O9-AIG-205

When Someone You Love Suffers from Posttraumatic Stress

When Someone You Love Suffers from Posttraumatic Stress

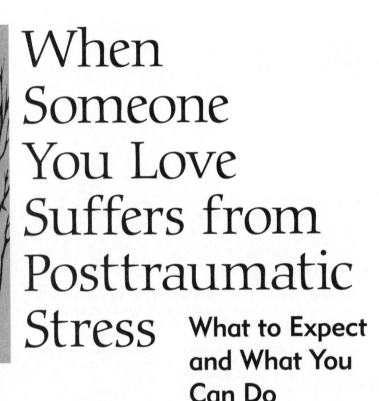

What to Expect and What You Can Do

Claudia Zayfert, PhD
Jason C. DeViva, PhD

THE GUILFORD PRESS
New York   London

© 2011 The Guilford Press
A Division of Guilford Publications, Inc.
72 Spring Street, New York, NY 10012
www.guilford.com

All rights reserved

The information in this volume is not intended as a substitute for
consultation with healthcare professionals. Each individual's health
concerns should be evaluated by a qualified professional.

Except as indicated, no part of this book may be reproduced, translated,
stored in a retrieval system, or transmitted, in any form or by any
means, electronic, mechanical, photocopying, microfilming, recording,
or otherwise, without written permission from the publisher.

Printed in the United States of America

This book is printed on acid-free paper.

Last digit is print number: 9   8   7   6   5   4   3   2   1

Library of Congress Cataloging-in-Publication Data

Zayfert, Claudia.
    When someone you love suffers from posttraumatic stress : what to
expect and what you can do / Claudia Zayfert, Jason C. DeViva.
        p.   cm.
    Includes bibliographical references and index.
    ISBN 978-1-60918-196-3 (hardcover) — ISBN 978-1-60918-065-2
(pbk.)
    1. Post-traumatic stress disorder—Popular works.   I. DeViva,
Jason C.   II. Title.
    RC552.P67Z39 2011
    616.85 21—dc22
    2011000368

To my mother, Ada, for being there through this
—C. Z.

To my parents, for always believing in me;
to my wife, for her unquestioning support;
and to the wives and partners of the CT NG
AVCRAD, for telling me how things really are
instead of listening quietly
—J. C. D.

Acknowledgments

We would like to acknowledge all the people who contributed to the writing of this book. First and foremost, we thank our patients and those who love them and support them during treatment for having the courage to trust us with their stories and their recovery. Without the work that patients and their loved ones have been willing to do, we simply would not have been able to write this book. We are immensely grateful to our editors at The Guilford Press: Kitty Moore, whose vision made this book possible, and Christine Benton, whose insightful and meticulous editing helped us bring it to life. Their inspiration, guidance, and diligent feedback helped shape our ideas and experiences and sharpen our focus on the needs of the loved ones who stand, quiet and steadfast, beside trauma survivors everywhere.

Many mentors and colleagues have influenced our thinking on trauma and its effects on those around the survivor, and contributed to our professional development over the years. We would like to acknowledge Dharm Bains, Carolyn Black Becker, Bill Bloem, Scott Driesenga, Candace Monson, Jacqueline Persons, Paula Schnurr, Kelly Bemis Vitousek, and VA Connecticut's OEF/OIF Outreach and Clinical Team. We are also grateful to all the trauma survivors, veterans, family members, and clinicians who have given us feedback in our clinical practice and at the various workshops and outreach talks we have presented over the years.

Finally, we express our deepest gratitude to *our* loved ones, Chris Wilcox and Kimberly DeViva, for supporting us as we labored on this book.

Contents

PART III

Coping with Specific Traumas

PART IV

Putting Your Lives Back Together

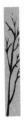

Introduction

Joe could not understand why he never saw his brother, Tom, anymore. They had been close all their lives and lived only a 45-minute freeway ride apart. Since the car accident last May, Tom had visited less and less frequently. He used to drive up to see Joe every weekend. After the crash, he was making it up only once a month. Then Joe noticed Tom wasn't making the trip at all. The times when Joe drove to visit his brother, Tom never seemed happy to have someone else in his house; in fact, it seemed to Joe that Tom hardly left home at all. It was like his brother, his best friend, was pulling away from him; and worse, because of all the negativity coming from Tom, Joe could sense himself pulling away, too. It didn't make sense to Joe; after all, when the other car slammed into Tom's, all his airbags had deployed correctly. Even though both cars were totaled and the other driver had to be pulled out of the wreckage, Tom had walked away from the accident with only a bump on the head. Why would the accident bother him so much?

Juan knew that after his wife, Estelle, had been attacked and almost raped downtown she would be different. He really thought he was trying his best to give her space and not push her back into her normal life. But sometimes he wasn't sure he was doing the right thing. Was he "enabling," like they said in Alcoholics Anonymous? And now that he thought of it, Estelle was drinking a lot more than she had before she was attacked. She wasn't doing it to get drunk, just to get to sleep at night, but still, Juan was concerned about her health.

Jenny and the entire family were at the airport to welcome her husband, Marcus, home from Iraq. He was happy to see everyone at first, but that seemed to wear off pretty quickly. He was irritable and jumpy all the time, and couldn't stand any noises or loud voices. It seemed like the harder Jenny tried to reach out to him, the more he pulled back. And it wasn't just her; he didn't seem to want anything to do with anyone. In the fall, their eldest daughter, Marion, was so concerned about him that she didn't want to go back to school for her junior year of college. Jenny finally convinced her to return, but when they made the trip Marcus, who usually drove her and all her stuff up to school, stayed home.

If someone you care about has been through something traumatic, the preceding stories probably sound familiar to you. You may have picked up this book because someone you care about suffered a terrible event and was diagnosed with posttraumatic stress disorder (PTSD), and you want to know more about this diagnosis and what it means for your loved one and her future. Alternatively, someone important in your life may have withdrawn from you and the rest of the world after something awful happened to him, and you want to do what you can to make sure he gets help. Or you may have watched someone you love endure a traumatic event, and even though everything seems okay so far, you're concerned about what to expect.

Most people don't know what makes an event traumatic or how trauma can affect the survivor's life. When you first learned about what happened to your loved one, you probably felt sad and angry that someone you care about had endured something terrible. You may also have felt frightened that he had been endangered and then relieved when he survived. Perhaps you thought that once it was all over everything would go back to normal. Many people do pick up the pieces and get back to their lives quickly after traumatic events, but for some, life is changed irrevocably and they feel stuck, unable to move forward. When things didn't go back to the way they were, you probably felt confused, and maybe even angry at the survivor for not "getting over it" or "moving on." In fact, one of the most common questions that family members ask us is "Will she always be this way?"

Survivors of traumatic events such as physical or sexual assaults, combat deployments, accidents, or natural disasters can experience a variety of problems. As recently as 40 years ago, little was known about how survivors of traumatic stress are affected by their experiences. Since that time there has been a tremendous amount of research on psychological trauma, greatly expanding our knowledge of its effects on the lives of survivors. This research has led to the development of effective treatments that can help survivors of traumatic events live healthier and more satisfying lives. In our work as clinical psychologists, we have used these treatments to help countless trauma survivors recover from posttraumatic stress and move forward in their lives. Our experience has shown us that treatment can work. It offers hope for many trauma survivors who have otherwise felt stuck trying to cope on their own.

We have also come to realize that although a wide range of information and services is available to help trauma survivors, the difficulties faced by the friends and family of those survivors are often overlooked. There are books, pamphlets, websites, and even DVDs for survivors of trauma, but few resources for the people in their lives who are indirectly yet seriously affected by the trauma. Loved ones and friends of trauma survivors often read materials written for the survivor, which can be informative but don't tell them much about what they can expect or do for themselves. In the course of our contact with the husbands, wives, partners, sons, daughters, parents, and friends of our patients we have found that they invariably have many questions about trauma and its effects and about what they can expect. Although most want to know what they can do to help their loved ones, frequently we see signs that they also are in need of help for themselves. Traumatic stress can be a source of anguish, frustration, sadness, and fatigue in loved ones as well as trauma survivors. Therefore, our main reason for writing this book is to fill a gap and offer help specifically for family and friends of trauma survivors who want to understand the changes in their loved one *and* take better care of themselves. Of course, we hope that in offering this guidance and support we'll also help those who have experienced trauma. Research has shown that when survivors of trauma have good social support, their chances of recovery improve. If family members and friends understand the effects of trauma and feel equipped to take care of themselves, they will be better able to help their loved ones, which could speed the recovery of the trauma survivor. *By helping to strengthen the coping resources of the important people in our patients' lives, we can bolster the support provided to our patients so they have a greater chance of healing.*

Hope for Healing, Hope for Change

The most important information we can offer about the effects of trauma on you and your loved one is this: *It doesn't have to be this way.* There are things you can do to help yourself and to make your life better. There are things you can do to improve your relationship with the trauma survivor in your life. There are things you can do to help the survivor heal. We wrote this book to guide you in doing these things.

We hope that by the end of this book you will realize that you are not alone in caring about someone who has been traumatized. Many loved ones of trauma survivors share your feelings—helplessness, loneliness, frustration, sadness, and anger may be intermingled with love, empathy, and caring. It is common and perfectly normal to experience such a complicated mix of feelings. We hope this book will help you take care of yourself and make sure your needs are met while you care for the trauma survivor in your life. And we hope that you will gain knowledge about what you can do to help yourself and your loved one to live healthy, meaningful lives.

What's in This Book?

This book has four parts. In the first section, we describe the effects of trauma on the survivor and on the people around him. We want to help you understand all the ways that the trauma has affected your life, as well as all the different ways it has touched your loved one. We talk about how the effects of trauma can change over time. We also outline the treatment options available to your loved one and provide guidance for how to seek professional help.

In the second section, we talk about what you can do to help yourself and help the person in your life who has been traumatized. We describe different ways in which you can take care of yourself and make sure your needs are met. We also talk about how to decide how much you are willing to do to help the trauma survivor in your life.

Finally, we describe methods of communicating with your loved one that will bring you closer together.

In the third section, we provide specific information relevant to two particular types of trauma: military trauma and sexual assault.

In the final section, we talk about the effects of trauma on intimate relationships as well as on children in your life. And we end the book by exploring an aspect of trauma that often is neglected—the positive changes that can occur in the trauma survivor and loved ones.

Real Stories of Hope and Change

We have tried to include as many stories as possible to illustrate the things we talk about. Each story is based on real people like you—people who struggled to cope with a loved one who was traumatized. Although we have changed the details about each family so that trauma survivors and their loved ones cannot be identified, we want you to keep in mind that these stories are based on real people and show their genuine feelings and thoughts. As you read, pay attention to similarities between your experiences and the stories in this book—we hope their examples will help you feel less alone. There are a lot of people out there who, like you, have seen someone they love experience trauma and then struggled to resume their lives. Their stories are an inspiration, and we hope their examples will help guide you to better days.

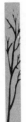

PART I

Understanding Posttraumatic Stress

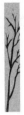

ONE

What It Feels Like to Live with a Trauma Survivor

Lucy was reaching the end of her willpower. It had been almost 6 months since Ed got back from his deployment to Afghanistan. He had been part of an engineering crew, and his reports back from Afghanistan had been generally okay. She knew he had been afraid the whole time, and knew that there were three or four events that really shook him up. But 6 months? When he first got back, he seemed relieved to be home, but then he started pulling away from her and the kids. He told her that his superiors in the National Guard had recommended they take about 30 days to transition back to civilian life, but he kept asking for more time. It didn't seem like he was trying to get a job or get out and be more active, and she was starting to lose her patience. How much more would she have to put up with?

Maggie and Ian were concerned about their daughter, Tess, but didn't know what to do. Tess had been sexually assaulted by three men while she was away at college. Maggie and Ian had watched their usually outgoing and happy girl slowly recede into a shell, and it didn't seem like there was anything they could do to help. She had returned to school, but her grades had dropped and she didn't seem to be taking care of herself. They tried to visit as often as they could, but she didn't seem interested in spending time with anyone. They had even tried calling the college's health center on their own, but the person on the phone told them there was nothing the college could do if Tess didn't come in on her own. Maggie and Ian wanted to take care of their daughter but they felt helpless.

Juan was tired all day but couldn't sleep at night. It didn't help that most nights Estelle either was tossing and turning or she was not in the bed at all. But even when the bedroom was quiet, he would lie awake at night and worry. Would their marriage always be like this? Could it ever go back to the way it was? Worst of all, he couldn't stop blaming himself for all of it. He was supposed to protect his wife; if he had been there, she wouldn't have been attacked. And he should know what to do now to help her. But everything he said or did seemed to backfire and just make Estelle either angrier or sadder.

When your loved one is traumatized, the experience and your loved one's reactions to it can affect your life and your relationship—your lives together—in many ways. You probably have a lot of unanswered questions and may feel confused, frustrated, even frightened by what the future might hold. Can you identify with any of the following responses that we often see in the loved ones of survivors?

"It doesn't make sense."

Loved ones often feel a sense of **confusion** about the trauma survivor's response to the situation. As noted earlier, Joe couldn't understand why Tom was so affected by the car crash. It didn't make sense to him that Tom could be that bothered by a crash he had walked away from. Joe thought he should have been relieved to come home. Maureen felt similar confusion when her husband, Ralph, returned from a deployment to Bosnia in 1997. She could understand how he might have been bothered by the terrible things he saw, but it made no sense to her that he didn't just get over it and move on with his life. And why wouldn't he talk about what happened when he was there? She could take it. After all, she had grown up in a big city, with all sorts of bad things happening all the time.

Friends and family of trauma survivors often cannot understand why their loved one can't seem to "get over" an incident from the past, even one that was traumatic. They may have little understanding of what actually happened because the survivor is not willing to talk about the trauma. They may not understand why his difficulties won't go away and might even get worse over time.

"I never know who will show up."

Friends and loved ones of survivors of trauma often report that they **can never predict** what sort of mood the survivor will be in from one minute to the next. Susan, whose husband, Jerry, had served in the Gulf War, said that his mood changed almost from minute to minute. She had no way to know what would affect him: "Sometimes when we are out with friends, Jerry is talkative and sociable. Other times, he stays in a corner or outside and asks me to leave after just a few minutes. I never know who will show up." She used go along with whatever he was up for, but after a while she became frustrated at not seeing their friends, so she would drive him home and then return to the gathering by herself. This meant they spent less time together, and she was not sharing good times with him. Susan was feeling more and more distant from Jerry.

At times there may be clear causes, or "triggers," of the trauma survivor's angry, irritable, or isolating mood. For example, Susan knew that if Jerry saw a movie about war he would probably be in a bad mood for the rest of the day. Similarly, Jenny knew that no matter what sort of mood Marcus was in when they got to a family function, if someone asked him about his time in Iraq he would suddenly become quiet and sad. At other times, there may be no clear trigger for the irritability or isolation. It seemed to Juan that sometimes Estelle would wake up in a bad mood. She would start the day angry or unresponsive, before anything had even happened. If the trauma survivor in your life seems to get upset out of the blue, for no clear reason that you can see, you may feel that you can't predict what sort of mood he will be in from one minute to the next.

"I'm walking on eggshells."

Trauma survivors often show extreme emotional sensitivity, so that even little things can upset them. As a result, family members often find themselves "tiptoeing around" in an **effort to cause the survivor as little distress as possible.** To avoid upsetting the survivor, they try not to burden her with requests, chores, or phone calls. They also may try to be very careful about what they say and how they say it because they don't want to suffer the consequences of having made their loved one angry. One man described this as "walking on eggshells" because he had to be so careful around his wife. Marion quickly learned that talking about the economy, the news, or her hopes and dreams about college upset her father, Marcus. So she learned to focus their conversations on sports and to choose her words carefully.

Perhaps the most unfortunate consequence of "walking on eggshells" is that the family member takes over most of the household chores and duties. Jeff, whose wife, Emily, had been in a bad car accident, realized in the months after the crash that paying the bills got Emily agitated for what seemed like days. So he gradually started paying all of the bills in addition to his other chores. When 6 months had passed since the crash, Jeff also was cleaning everything in the house and maintaining the cars. As much as he cared for Emily and wanted her to feel better, he started to resent the fact that he was carrying the entire burden of running the house.

"He gets angry at the drop of a hat. I can't take it anymore."

Loved ones can find it challenging to cope with the moodiness and anger that some trauma survivors display on a daily basis. They often talk about the **frustration and powerlessness** they feel. Instead of withdrawing and walking on eggshells around the trauma survivor, some family and friends may do just the opposite and interact with the survivor in aggressive ways. You may have noticed that the trauma survivor in your life can get angry very quickly. If the survivor feels trapped and does not think she has any other way to maintain a sense of control in her life, aggression may be the only way she can feel powerful. It is difficult to stay calm when someone is yelling at you, so you may have fallen into a similar pattern of aggression when responding to the survivor. Wanda's husband, Nadim, had been mugged and beaten one summer night. By winter he had become sullen and withdrawn. To Wanda, he seemed to communicate only by yelling at her.

Eventually, she had had enough and started yelling back. On two separate occasions, neighbors had called the police after hearing shouting and crashing sounds from their apartment.

"What possibly could have happened?"

You might not know exactly what happened to the trauma survivor in your life, and that might make it really hard to understand how she is being affected by the trauma. When the trauma survivor does not confide in you, you may feel **distrusted, hurt, and frustrated**. For example, Sean knew that his sister, Kate, had been working at the factory when one of the massive steam-heaters blew and a lot of people were burned. But the news reports had been vague as to how badly they were hurt. Kate had been on the other side of the factory at the time but somehow ended up with minor burns. When Sean called to ask her what had happened, she only stammered, "I tried to help" and then hung up the phone. In the two months since then, she had not been back to work and had hardly spoken to anyone. Sean couldn't make sense of what she was going through; he kept asking himself, "What possibly could have happened?"

You may be wondering the same thing. Trauma survivors often are reluctant to talk about what they experienced. The people who care about them are left wondering what they went through and why it bothers them so much. You may even have directly asked the survivor to tell you what happened, only to have him refuse to talk about it. This may have left you not only confused about the trauma but also struggling to understand why he wouldn't trust you enough to share what happened. This can be a frustrating process. You want to help and to understand, but the survivor seems totally unwilling to open up and you feel left in the dark.

"I don't want to know!"

Loved ones often feel **horrified** by the events the survivor experienced. When Marcus communicated with Jenny while he was in Iraq, he updated her on the kinds of things his unit was doing. They were involved in some combat operations but often worked with civilians.

One of the things Marcus told Jenny he enjoyed most was interacting with local families, especially the children. They made him think of his own family, and he felt more connected to the Iraqis. But then Marcus seemed to stop talking about civilians. He mentioned at one point that there had been a blast in a marketplace but didn't give a lot of detail. His sudden reluctance to share his experiences with Jenny confused her. She wanted to ask him what had happened in that explosion, but she realized that she was scared to hear the answer. What if children had been hurt or killed? She couldn't bear the idea of young people being involved in a war. She had a hard time imagining her husband, with two beautiful kids of his own, seeing children injured or killed. She found herself dreading calls from Marcus and hoping he wouldn't talk about what was happening over there because she was not sure she could handle it. Whenever he did talk about specific events, she would think to herself, "I don't want to know! Don't tell me!"

You may want desperately to help the trauma survivor in your life, but you also may want to remain in the dark about what he went through. Hearing about very distressing events, especially when they happened to someone you care about, can cause you to think more about those events than you otherwise might have. You also might struggle with anger, sadness, and helplessness when you think about exactly what happened to your loved one. You might find yourself, as Jenny had, thinking that you really don't want to know what happened to the person you care about. You may hope that she doesn't try to tell you. Juan knew from her bruises that Estelle had been physically attacked during the assault. Images of two men grabbing and punching her came into his mind when he least expected it, and he found them very upsetting. He felt horrible when he thought about his wife, who would never hurt a fly, suffering at the hands of complete strangers. When the police came to ask Estelle some follow-up questions, Juan wanted to stay with her for support. But he found it too hard and realized he didn't want to hear the details about what happened that night.

"What am I doing wrong?"

When the loved ones of trauma survivors do not know about the effects of trauma, they may blame themselves for the survivor's behavior. This can lead to feelings of **guilt**. When her boyfriend Charlie came back from Afghanistan, Meagan knew from what she saw on TV that he would probably have nightmares and flashbacks. But no one told her that survivors of trauma often avoid other people and have difficulty experiencing feelings like love or happiness. As Charlie withdrew and seemed to have no emotional response to her, she started to wonder why. This didn't seem related to his flashbacks so she started to wonder whether she was doing or saying something to drive him away. As much as she tried to draw him closer, he never seemed to respond to her with the love he showed her before his deployment. She asked herself over and over, "What am I doing wrong?"

Not knowing the extent of trauma's effects, Meagan did what many loved ones of trauma survivors do. She assumed Charlie's behavior was the result of something she was doing, so she tried to fix it. This often led to her feeling frustrated and hopeless; no matter what she changed or tried, Meagan couldn't get Charlie to act the way he had before he was deployed. After a few months, Meagan left Charlie, less because of how he treated her than because of how she thought he felt about her. You may feel so confused about changes in the trauma survivor that you blame yourself for the problems that he is having now. Unfortunately, blaming yourself not only leads to feeling guilty for something you did not do but also makes you think it is your responsibility to change the survivor, which places an almost impossible burden on you.

"We're not as close as we used to be."

Trauma survivors often isolate themselves from their loved ones. As a result, even their closest family and friends feel as though they have grown worlds apart from the survivor. This **loss of intimacy** can be devastating for loved ones. Despite the fact that he spent most of his free time at his brother's house, Joe didn't feel close to Tom. It seemed like they barely talked even when they were together. Tom didn't seem comfortable opening up anymore. This was hard for Joe to take. As brothers, they had always been each other's best friend, and had always told each other everything. It felt weird that Tom never came up to visit him, even though Joe was willing to drive to see Tom at a moment's notice. Joe felt like the relationship had become a one-way street.

Even if the trauma survivor doesn't completely isolate herself from her loved ones, her intimate relationships may suffer. A spouse may become more distant, a son may interact less with his father, or, as in the case of Joe and Tom, one brother may no longer trust in and open up to the other. Many trauma survivors say they can feel alone even in a room full of people. Loved ones and family are often aware of the trauma survivor's detachment, and they may even feel the same way themselves. Even if you see the trauma survivor often or live with her, you may feel as though the two of you have lost the intimacy you once had.

"We don't see anyone anymore."

The **isolation** of trauma survivors can gradually shrink the worlds of those who care about them. This is especially the case for family members who live with trauma survivors or spend a lot of time with them. When the two brothers were invited to family events, Tom would call Joe and ask him to come spend the day at his house. Joe would be put in the position of either not visiting with family or refusing to see his brother. He started to feel like whatever he did would be wrong. Similarly, Marion knew her father got very uncomfortable when people asked him about Iraq. She felt terrible when Marcus left family gatherings alone, so she started going home with him so he would have company. She was spending much less time with her cousins and grandparents than she would like in order to make sure her father wasn't alone.

In the case of couples such as Juan and Estelle, the isolation of the survivor can result in isolation of the partner. The survivor avoids activities that the couple usually did together, and the partner, unaccustomed to doing those things alone, also stops participating in those activities. Juan realized that they saw fewer and fewer of their friends as a result of Estelle's desire to avoid social gatherings. Juan was concerned about Estelle and did not like leaving her home alone. As a result, he soon lost contact with most of his friends. When he complained to Estelle, "We don't see anyone anymore," she seemed completely unconcerned.

"I'm not getting my sleep."

Loved ones of trauma survivors may suffer from **sleep disruption.** If you share a bed with a trauma survivor, chances are you have noticed that he doesn't sleep well. This may be affecting your sleep, too. You may wake up during the night when your loved one tosses and turns. If the trauma survivor has nightmares, you may wake up when she moves around or makes noise. Jenny was startled out of a sound sleep when Marcus cried out next to her. She asked him what was wrong, but he just kept yelling. When she couldn't understand what he was saying and he didn't respond to her, she realized he was asleep and having a bad dream. The next morning he didn't remember dreaming at all.

Your sleep may be disrupted by the trauma survivor even if you don't share a bed because the survivor may have nighttime habits or routines that keep you awake. Keith and Ellie's son, Todd, stayed with them after he returned from Iraq while he was trying to find a job. Todd didn't feel safe at night and usually stayed up all night to watch the house. He also watched TV all night to distract himself from bad thoughts that bothered him when the house was quiet. The house was small, so Todd's nighttime activity disturbed Ellie's sleep. Ellie and Keith struggled with Todd to try to find a compromise that would allow them all to get the rest they needed.

"When is it my time?"

Often, family members of trauma survivors sacrifice their own goals, enjoyment, and friendships to accommodate the survivor. This can lead to feelings of **resentment**. After Ed returned from Afghanistan he was unable to work due to his symptoms, so his wife, Lucy, took a second job so they wouldn't lose their home. Before the accident at work, Sandy and Gary had agreed that in the spring semester Sandy would take night classes toward an advanced degree that could lead to a promotion at work. But with Gary unable to work due to injuries and nightmares, they couldn't afford the tuition for her degree program. So Sandy canceled her registration at the community college and put her plans off indefinitely.

The family and friends of survivors of trauma often feel hurt, angry, and disregarded as a result of the sacrifices they make. They may feel anger at society in general for not recognizing them, or resentful toward the survivor for missed opportunities in their own lives. It can seem unfair that the survivor receives sympathy and special treatment and is allowed time to recover, while the family member labors without recognition to keep the family afloat. The uncertainty about when they will have the chance to live their lives can lead to building resentment toward the trauma survivor. Loved ones may wonder, as did the wife of a combat veteran, "When is it my time?"

"This is not what I signed up for."

Changes in the trauma survivor often alter the nature of her relationships with her loved ones, leading loved ones to feel a sense of **disappointment and loss**. When Juan had first met Estelle, she loved to be around people, whether it was old friends or people she had just met. She was perpetually busy, and had many activities and interests. One of the things Juan loved most about her was her smile, which always brightened his day. After the assault, this all seemed to change. She no longer wanted to be around other people, especially strangers, and she hardly ever smiled anymore. She no longer engaged in the activities she used to enjoy and only wanted to stay home. It seemed as if the woman he'd married had been taken away and replaced with someone different. On nights when Estelle refused to answer the phone, or asked him to go to the grocery store for her, he thought to himself, "This is not what I expected this marriage to be like. This is not what I signed up for."

You may have found yourself feeling like Juan. The changes in your loved one after the trauma may make it seem as if a different person has entered your life. The changes in the way you and your loved one interact may be so great that it feels like an entirely different relationship. You may notice yourself thinking that the relationship you're now in is not the relationship you had entered into, and the trauma seems to be the cause. You may be wondering whether the relationship is going to be this way forever, or whether it's a relationship you really want to be in.

But despite the changes, you may feel trapped. You may be the only person in the trauma survivor's life whom she trusts or with whom she feels comfortable. You might have considered leaving the relationship and then thought, "But if I leave, who will she have?" Wanda knew that, for all the yelling he did, Nadim felt closer to her than to anyone else. When he got scared at work or on the road he would always call her as soon as he could. They had been married for

8 years before he was mugged and beaten. Even though he seemed like a hollow shell of the man he had once been, she still loved him and couldn't bear the thought of leaving him when he was at his worst and needed her most.

What You May Feel

As someone who loves a trauma survivor, you may feel many complex emotions. Sometimes you may be overwhelmed by one very intense feeling. In other instances, you may feel several different emotions or even have two "opposite" feelings at the same time. You might even have difficulty recognizing what you're feeling. Your emotions can be intense and may seem to change from one minute to the next. The many different and sometimes conflicting feelings can be confusing and overwhelming.

Watching someone you care about struggle after trauma can be difficult. It's common to **worry or feel anxiety** when you think about the trauma survivor in your life. Joe worried constantly about Tom and wondered whether the changes in his brother were temporary or permanent. Juan's main fear concerning Estelle was about the consequences of her drinking. He fell asleep each night thinking she might be drinking herself to death. Bob's son, Wayne, who had served in the Gulf War, lived several states away. Wayne hated the phone, so they kept in touch mostly over the Internet. Bob noticed that Wayne's e-mail and blog posts had an increasingly angry tone. To Bob it sounded like Wayne was looking for a reason to be violent. He feared that Wayne might really hurt someone, be thrown in jail, or be badly hurt himself.

Family and friends also may feel **sadness** about the effects of trauma on their loved ones. As we discuss in Chapter 2, the effects of trauma can be chronic and at times debilitating. As Jenny watched her husband slowly withdraw from life, she felt very sad about what Marcus was going through and the losses he was experiencing. As Estelle's husband, Juan not only witnessed his wife's suffering but also felt his own sense of loss due to what was missing from his life. They did not go out anymore and barely saw their friends. Though he himself had not been traumatized, Juan also experienced losses due to Estelle's trauma.

Friends and loved ones of trauma survivors almost always want to do whatever they can to help. They may go out of their way to call or check in on the trauma survivor, offer to talk, or suggest things to help him feel better. They also may offer to help him find professional help and even go with him to treatment. As we discuss in Chapter 3, however, it is very difficult to make another person change. Often loved ones' efforts to help are not effective. In some cases the survivor may respond to offers of help by withdrawing even more. As a result, family and friends can often feel **helpless**, as if nothing they do makes a difference. Bob, whose son Wayne lived far from him, tried to call Wayne several times a week, but no matter what message he left on the answering machine, Wayne never called him back. When Joe couldn't get Tom to answer his phone, he would stop by his house. Even when Joe was physically present in the room, Tom would not interact with him any more than he had to. They would simply sit together and watch TV. Joe often found himself wanting to stop calling and give up on his brother.

Joe also found himself struggling not to get mad at Tom. He found himself thinking, "Don't you see how hard I'm trying?" His helplessness had slowly shifted to **anger** at his brother. Loved ones and friends of trauma survivors can feel angry for a number of reasons. For example, Joe became frustrated with Tom's unresponsiveness to his attempts to help. Juan felt angry at Estelle because he thought her reactions to the assault had taken away many of the things they loved. At times he noticed himself blaming her for having bad dreams or refusing to do things. After Wallace's wife, Maria, returned from deployment to Afghanistan she snapped at him over little things and often made belittling remarks about his job and the things that he worried about. She told him that if he had been to war such minor things wouldn't bother him. When Wallace later heard her talking on the phone in a friendly tone to soldiers she had served with, he became angry at how Maria treated him.

You also may have noticed yourself feeling angry at those who were responsible for the trauma that hurt your loved one. As angry as Wallace was at Maria, he was even angrier at the National Guard. Why did they have to send her over? Shouldn't they have let a married person stay home with her family and sent someone else? And why weren't they taking care of her now? Lea had never worried about her son, Kip, working at the mall until he was assaulted and robbed behind the store where he worked. She couldn't believe that something like that could happen in broad daylight. The mall owners should have paid closer attention to what was occurring on their property. There should have been cameras and security guards nearby who could have heard Kip calling for help.

As Joe started to drift away from Tom, he began to feel **guilty**. He thought that he should do all that he could to help his brother and anything less than 100% effort was letting his brother down and abandoning him. Similarly, as soon as Juan started blaming Estelle for the decline of their social life, he became angry at himself. It's not her fault, he told himself; what right do you have to judge? Marion started to feel guilty for calling her father, Marcus, on the phone from college when it was clear he didn't want to talk. After all, she reasoned, he had served his country and fought for her freedom. Hadn't he earned some time to readjust?

Like trauma survivors, families and loved ones can feel a range of emotions. Often, however, family and loved ones think that they are not allowed to feel what they are feeling. You may believe you don't deserve to complain because you were not the one who was traumatized. You also may be reluctant to express your concerns to the trauma survivor for fear he will react intensely. If you try to convey your concerns to the survivor and offer to help, your attempt to reach out may be met with anger, rejection, or indifference.

You have every right to feel the way you feel. Your emotions are neither right nor wrong; they are understandable responses to the experience of living with a trauma survivor. Do not judge yourself negatively for being confused, afraid, or angry. Allow yourself to feel whatever you are feeling. Do not try to escape or suppress your emotions. Instead, accept them and focus on taking care of yourself. In Chapter 6, we talk more about how to manage your feelings and act constructively to make sure your own needs are met. But first, let's look at how and why trauma has affected your loved one and what you can expect in the future.

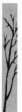

TWO

How Trauma Affects Survivors

Joe was getting angrier and angrier at his brother. Tom had just about stopped leaving the house and didn't like to talk to anyone, even Joe. Joe could understand why Tom might be afraid of cars— but people? Joe was so frustrated that once he even yelled at Tom that it was only a car accident, that he should just get over it. This turned out to be a bad move. Tom just got up and went into his room and didn't come out again until Joe left an hour later.

Lucy thought that Ed would have flashbacks and nightmares when he got back from Afghanistan, but that never happened. She thought he might be on guard a lot, because she saw that on TV, and that definitely happened. He was so focused on watching everyone when they went out that she could see him sweating in a restaurant. She hadn't expected all the moving around in his sleep, and she definitely hadn't expected all the dangerous things he was doing. Getting into fights, driving fast, talking about skydiving—was that supposed to happen?

Andy was amazed they had survived the tornado. The house would need a new roof (the winds had ripped it clean off), but they had been okay in the basement. It definitely got scary when the neighbors' wheelbarrow came crashing through the bulkhead, and he and Lilly had been pretty sure they had heard the roof come off. But the whole thing hadn't lasted more than 10 minutes. Lilly had seemed to take it pretty hard. She hadn't slept a wink in the 2 months since the tornado, and she was constantly snappy. A few times she had startled, just about jumped out of her skin, and some of those times Andy couldn't even figure out what she was jumping at. What was with her? As far as he was concerned, they were lucky to be alive.

Many trauma survivors who come to us for help ask us to educate their family members about the effects of trauma. Survivors often have difficulty explaining the complexities of posttraumatic stress, especially when they're just learning about it for the first time themselves: "I tried to explain it, but it all came out wrong and she just ended up more confused than before. Can she come in and hear you say it?" The survivor also may want to convey to his loved one that his behavior has an understandable cause and is not a sign of who he really is: "Can you tell her that I snap at her because I'm stressed? Can you tell her that it's not her fault?"

Trauma survivors usually know they've experienced something bad and recognize that it's causing difficulty in their lives. They realize that some symptoms, such as nightmares, are connected to their traumatic experiences, yet they may have difficulty recognizing this connection for other symptoms, such as poor sleep, depression, irritability, trouble concentrating, or feeling detached from others. Estelle was aware that her anxiety and avoidance of public places were connected to the assault. She did not realize, however, that the assault was responsible for her feeling emotionally disconnected from Juan. Ed was aware that he had had a "short fuse" since returning from Afghanistan, but he didn't realize how this was related to his war experiences. Jake realized that he had been highly uncomfortable around men his entire life, but he didn't connect this to having been molested as a child by his uncle. Ever since she was assaulted, Sarah had trouble concentrating at work and was forgetful, irritable, and jumpy, but she didn't realize how the assault might be related to these problems.

Puzzling changes in your loved one's mood, personality, or preferences have probably left you feeling confused, afraid, and frustrated. This confusion leads some loved ones of trauma survivors to blame themselves for the changes in the survivor. In Chapter 1 we described how Meagan left Charlie after trying unsuccessfully to change whatever she was doing to make Charlie withdraw from her after he got back from Afghanistan. Understanding how traumatic events can affect the person who lives through them will help you avoid blaming yourself and, more important, inform you about what can change if the survivor in your life gets help.

Trauma and Stress

A trauma is a type of stressful event. It can be helpful to think of stressful events on a continuum, with the least intense on one end and the most severe on the other. On one end of the continuum are daily hassles, the little things that can be irritating, frustrating, or worrisome—such as getting caught in traffic, forgetting to pay a bill, or missing your bus so that you are late to work. Further along the continuum are moderate stressors. These are things that are not out of the ordinary but are more worrisome and difficult than daily hassles. Examples include a big fight with your spouse, finding out a child is failing at school, or needing to repair all the plumbing in a bathroom. Major stressors usually occur less frequently than moderate stressors and are more severe. The death of someone very close to you, divorce, loss of a job, and a debilitating medical problem are examples of major stressors.

Traumatic events are at the far end of the spectrum. Typically these are dangerous events, and often they are experienced firsthand. As the event is happening, the person going through it may have to struggle to stay alive or help others survive. Traumatic events place a great strain on those who endure them. They typically are distinguished from other stressors by the perception of serious danger and the urge to fight or run for one's life. Reactions to trauma typically include intense fear, helplessness, or horror. Survivors often also describe a sense of shock, numbness, or disbelief. These reactions can be immediate, although sometimes they are delayed. After the trauma, the person also may develop feelings of intense guilt, shame, anger, or grief that can magnify and perpetuate her distress.

Often, traumatic events involve serious harm, a violation of the body, or actual death. Marcus was injured when a bomb exploded near him. Estelle was physically beaten and sexually assaulted by the two men who attacked her. Pamela was molested by a babysitter on multiple occasions when she was 10 years old. Although he did not inflict a physical injury or even threaten her with harm, she felt her body had been violated. She felt frightened and powerless when it was happening, and for years afterward she was plagued by guilt and shame.

It is important to note that a person does not have to be the one injured to be traumatized by an event. For example, on three occasions during his deployment Marcus watched men die from bullets and explosions, although he was unharmed. After his accident, Tom saw that the driver of the other car appeared seriously injured. He watched as paramedics attended to the victim and whisked him away by ambulance with sirens blaring. Neither Marcus nor Tom was badly hurt, but each witnessed others seriously injured or dying, which can be traumatic.

Events also can be traumatic if they include a serious threat of harm. Huang and his wife, Anne, were held up at gunpoint. The robbery lasted less than two minutes, but the whole time Huang had a gun pressed against his forehead and he believed that he was going to die. From Huang's perspective, there was a serious threat of harm. Marcus's platoon was involved in several firefights in which enemy soldiers were attacking them. Neither Marcus nor his buddies were hurt, but the bullets flying near them were definitely a serious threat. The threat need not involve weapons and often can be indirect. Tabitha's father was an alcoholic who frequently came home drunk, yelling at her and her mother, calling them names, throwing and breaking things in the home. Although he never specifically threatened to harm her, she grew up feeling terrorized. Similarly, Violet had been married to a controlling and emotionally abusive man for 4 years. He was large and intimidating. His constant yelling together with the lack of control over her life made Violet feel trapped and unsafe.

Sometimes the trauma survivor may not experience the event firsthand, but he may witness the aftermath. For example, Marcus was affected not only by witnessing men being shot but also by seeing the remains of soldiers who had been blown up when their vehicle was struck by a suicide bomber. He arrived two hours after the blast, but he saw the effects of the bomb close up and was horrified. Dennis lived in the town next to Andy and Lilly's community, where the tornado touched down. When he went with members of his church to help the next day, he was stunned by the total destruction just 15 miles from where he lived.

Some trauma survivors haven't even directly witnessed an event but have learned that something terrible happened to someone close to them. Jeremy was awakened by a phone call in the middle of the night informing him that his son had been killed when his motorcycle was hit by a truck. Mary learned that her elderly mother had been brutally murdered by home invaders. Alicia's son was shot by a man who charged into his classroom at school and began randomly shooting students. Alicia's son died from his injuries in the hospital a week later. Alicia, like Mary and many other family members of homicide victims, was severely traumatized by this loss.

Many different events can be experienced as traumatic. Some examples are:

- Being caught in a natural disaster, such as a hurricane, tornado, or earthquake
- Being threatened with a gun, knife, or other weapon
- Being in a serious motor vehicle accident
- Being physically assaulted or beaten
- Being forced to have sexual contact against your will
- Being in a war zone or witnessing the results of combat or terrorist attacks
- Being in a serious accident at work or during recreational activity
- Being kidnapped or held against your will
- Being physically or sexually abused or watching others be abused
- Being involved in rescuing others from dangerous situations or recovering bodies

At some point after finding out what happened to the trauma survivor in your life, you may have thought something like "How did this happen to him?" or "I never thought something like this would happen to someone I know!" In reality, although traumatic events happen far less often than daily hassles, they are not uncommon. Large-scale surveys tell us that at least 65% of Americans have experienced one or more traumatic events. To put this in perspective, imagine going to the movies. If the typical theater seats about 500 people, that means if a movie sells out, 325 people in that audience will have experienced a traumatic event at some point in life. **It is important to remember that the trauma survivor in your life is not unusual or strange because of what happened to him.**

But Why Are Some Things Traumatic to Some People?

After you read the three stories at the beginning of Chapter 1, you might have reacted like this: "I can see how a woman being attacked can be traumatic, and there are stories about soldiers and trauma all over the news. But a car crash? I've been in car accidents, and I was okay! And he wasn't even hurt!" One of the confusing aspects of trauma is that the same event can be traumatic to one person but not to another.

One key to determining whether an event will be experienced as traumatic is the intensity of emotions a person feels during or after the event. Two people may experience the same event involving threat of physical harm, and one may react with intense emotions whereas the other may not. For example, before going to Iraq, Marcus had never seen a dead body, let alone the remains of a person who was killed by a bomb. However, his buddy had worked for many years as an emergency medical technician (EMT) and witnessed many different scenes of violence, serious injury, and death in the course of his work. His EMT training prepared him to cope with such situations. When the two men came upon a dead body on the road, Marcus responded with intense horror whereas his buddy the medic took it in stride. Similarly, Marissa and Eli were on vacation in the Caribbean when a hurricane hit their island. They were sheltered in the main building of their resort and watched the wind blow several other buildings, including the beachfront cabana they had rented, into the ocean. The hurricane certainly involved a real threat of serious harm. However, Marissa was terrified the whole time and was sure they were going to die. Eli, on the other hand, was focused on his amazement at the power of nature and didn't feel scared. He thought the whole experience was pretty exciting. The hurricane was traumatic for Marissa, but not for Eli.

Interestingly, some people feel completely numb during such events, which is associated with having difficulties after the event. For example, Jake had been molested by his uncle many times when he was young. During each instance, Jake "checked out" in his own head and felt strangely numb to what was happening to him. Darren was deployed to Iraq during the initial invasion and was involved in intense fighting. He couldn't recall feeling fear during the invasion. Rather, he remembered feeling far away and strangely disconnected from what was happening to him, as if it wasn't real. Later in their lives, both Jake and Darren were troubled by intrusive memories and dreams about their experiences. They both struggled with feeling unsafe and needing to be constantly on guard for danger in many situations. They were prone to outbursts of anger that caused problems in their personal relationships. Despite these struggles, neither of them connected the problems they were having to the traumatic events, in part because they did not recall feeling bothered by them at the time they happened.

Why do some people experience certain emotions during stressful events and others do not? It is helpful to keep in mind that we do not choose the emotions we feel. Much of the time, emotions are not within our conscious control. Think, for example, of times when you've really wanted to remain calm. Have you always been able to? If you're like most people, there have been situations in your life when your emotions seemed to have "a mind of their own." Emotions are often knee-jerk reactions, and although we can exert some control over how we respond to them, emotions themselves are not planned or deliberate. It's important to understand that intense emotional reactions to a traumatic event are typical. They don't mean that the trauma survivor in your life is weak or abnormal. If you find yourself judging the trauma survivor for how she responded to the traumatic event, remember that she did not choose to be scared, angry, or sad about what happened. Something about the trauma triggered an intense emotional response in her, and she is struggling to deal with the aftereffects.

Try to resist putting yourself in your loved one's shoes. If you think about how you might have handled the situation, you may end up judging or second-guessing the trauma survivor. It's impossible to know how you would have reacted at that particular moment in that particular situation. Even if you had been in the same situation, there is no reason to assume that you and your loved one would have experienced the event in the same way. Judging the trauma survivor is not helpful and, in fact, can drive the survivor further away from you.

How Is the Trauma Affecting Your Loved One?

Traumatic events can have significant and lasting effects on those who experience them. Much like most other major events in our lives, traumatic events change us in both obvious and subtle ways. When most people think of the effects of trauma, the first thing that comes to mind is PTSD. We commonly think of PTSD as involving nightmares and flashbacks, yet many people have little understanding of why these intrusions occur and why they might continue after the event is long past. For most people, the hardest thing to understand about PTSD is why a person cannot just "get over it" and move on with life. Another aspect of PTSD that can be confusing is that not everyone with PTSD has nightmares or flashbacks. Two people both can be diagnosed with PTSD, but their symptoms can be quite different. This is because the core symptoms of PTSD—intrusions, hyperarousal, and avoidance, each discussed below—can be expressed in a variety of ways. In addition, there are many ways a person can be affected by a traumatic experience that do not meet the specific diagnostic criteria for PTSD but that nonetheless are very distressing and can seriously impair daily life. So let's look at the various ways that trauma can change a person's thoughts, emotional reactions, and behaviors and consider what keeps a person stuck reliving a past she so desperately would like to put behind her.

Reexperiencing Traumatic Events

A hallmark of PTSD is some form of intrusive reexperiencing of the trauma. Reexperiencing symptoms can interfere severely with the survivor's life. They are predominantly internal experiences (they happen inside the survivor's mind), so you may be unaware of when they are happening to your loved one. Trauma survivors can reexperience traumatic events in a variety of ways that can include any combination of thoughts, memories, and emotional distress, as well as bodily reactions and behaviors that may be observable to others.

Unwanted Memories

Trauma survivors often are bothered by **unwanted memories** of the events. Sometimes there is an obvious cue or "trigger" that prompts such thoughts. For example, movies about war remind Marcus of some of the longer firefights he experienced in Iraq. Sinead, who was sexually assaulted by a man with a heavy beard, is reminded of the assault when she sees a man with similar facial hair. At times, there may not be an obvious trigger of the unwanted memory, which can be confusing for both the trauma survivor and her loved one. Marcus's wife, Jenny, noticed that sometimes he suddenly became distant while watching something boring on television or relaxing after a long, busy day. When Marcus's mind was unoccupied, thoughts about Iraq would just pop up. Similarly, Joe's brother, Tom, found that violent images from the car crash popped into his head when he took a break from housecleaning on a Saturday morning.

Emotional and Physical Reactions to Reminders of the Trauma

One of the most confusing things for trauma survivors and their loved ones is that sometimes reminders of the traumatic event can suddenly trigger **intense emotional distress and/or bodily reactions** that may or may not be accompanied by memories of the trauma. A range of intense emotions, including fear, anger, guilt, shame, and sadness, can be triggered by reminders of a traumatic event even when the survivor is not aware that the reminders are connected to the event. After she was in a bus accident, Roxanne was extremely tense and anxious being a passenger in any vehicle, even though she had very little recollection of the accident itself. Sometimes she even experienced panic attacks and would insist that the driver slow down or let her out of the vehicle. Laura, who had been sexually assaulted several times throughout her life, stopped watching TV because she always ended up feeling intensely angry at the violence and the way women were being treated in TV shows. This caused problems in her marriage because her husband, Kevin, liked watching TV to wind down at night. Laura also had trouble being intimate with Kevin because she tensed up, or occasionally even flinched, when he touched her. Sometimes the only way she could be intimate was to pretend she was somewhere else, and Kevin felt hurt when he noticed she was so disconnected.

Mel's wife, Jane, who had been abused as a child, started crying during a news item about a kidnapped boy. Mel certainly had thought the story was sad, but Jane's reaction was far more intense than his. And he noticed that it lasted longer, as she still seemed to be sad the next day. Tara's twin sister, Caroline, was in a bad accident when Tara was 6 years old. Tara spent a lot of time in the hospital with her parents, visiting Caroline and feeling very confused, sad, and frightened.

Twenty years later Tara's husband, Craig, was in the hospital following minor surgery. When she walked in the door of the hospital to visit him, she suddenly felt intensely frightened and sad. Her heart started pounding, she became short of breath, queasy, and flushed, and she thought she would pass out. Not knowing why she felt this way, she left the hospital and went home to lie down, leaving Craig feeling hurt that she didn't visit. John, who had been molested by a priest as a child, made excuses to his wife to get out of going to her niece's wedding. The truth was he just couldn't cope with the intense shame and feeling of rage that overcame him whenever he walked through the door of a church. Marissa, who had watched a hurricane destroy the buildings that surrounded the shelter she was in, felt her spine crawl whenever it rained. During storms her heart rate went up, she broke out in a cold sweat, started breathing hard, and felt like she was going to pass out. The emotions and sensations triggered by trauma-related cues can be sudden, intense, and overwhelming. They may not make sense to the trauma survivor or those around him.

Flashbacks

For some trauma survivors, intrusive thoughts, sensations, and feelings can be so vivid and realistic that the survivor loses track of where he is at the time. He may feel as if the trauma is actually happening again. Steve had been pinned in a bunker for two hours by constant mortar and rocket fire while he was in a supposedly safe area of Iraq. The explosions at a fireworks show brought back intense memories of the bombing, and he felt as if it were happening again. He acted as if he were in danger and had to take cover. Such very intense memories are known as **flashbacks**. They are less common than other effects of trauma, but can be disconcerting to both the survivor and the people around him. During a flashback, a trauma survivor may be so immersed in reliving the event that she loses awareness that she is actually safe. She may even react to the perceived danger by fighting, screaming, or running from the situation. Standing in line at the supermarket behind a man who resembled one of her attackers, Estelle suddenly was reminded of the sexual assault. As the memory flooded back, she actually could smell the alcohol on the breath of the perpetrators and had the sensation that she was trapped. She left her cart where it was and ran away from the man and fled the store. This all happened so quickly that Juan was befuddled when he turned around and she wasn't there. He found her in the parking lot, huddled behind their car, shaking and crying.

Nightmares

Memories also can intrude during sleep in the form of **nightmares**. Trauma-related nightmares usually are more vivid and more intense than regular dreams. Some replay the actual traumatic event or parts of it. Freddie, who was in a serious accident at work, often awoke screaming from dreams in which he saw the forklift tumbling over and pinning him. Often the dream felt so real that his leg hurt and he had to feel it to make sure it wasn't broken again. Other nightmares are similar to the trauma, particularly in the emotional content, but don't exactly replay it. Trauma survivors also may experience "bad dreams" that are diffuse and scary, which they may or may not recall. For example, although Jane was beaten by her father, her dreams were of being chased in the dark with no way to escape.

Survivors are more likely to move around during trauma-related nightmares than you are when you dream. They may thrash or yell and may wake up terrified, in a "cold sweat." Their nightmares can be so graphic and disturbing that they can't go back to sleep. Eventually they may start to fear sleeping and be reluctant to go to bed. You may have sleep problems too, considering that many trauma survivors are not just restless but even combative during sleep.

Disruption of Daily Life

Regardless of how the survivor reexperiences the traumatic event, the memories, thoughts, dreams, and bodily reactions are often perceived as intrusions on daily life. These intrusions often interrupt activities for minutes, hours, or even an entire day. The emotional and physical reactions and ensuing efforts to suppress them can be physically draining. Trauma survivors often shift activities abruptly to escape memories, which can lead to social or work problems. For example, Sinead worked in a store. Whenever a man who resembled her assailant came in, she would panic and leave, sometimes not returning for several hours. After this happened a few times, her manager informed her that she was in danger of losing her job. Freddie's dreams were so disruptive to his sleep that frequently he could barely drag himself out of bed. He was so tired at work that he struggled to get through the day. His foreman let him know that he had noticed he was slow and made lots of mistakes.

You may have trouble understanding why your loved one persists in thinking about these awful things. You may wonder why he won't just let go of the past. The trauma survivor's brain learned to be prepared for danger. The intrusions are his brain's way of making sure he remembers what the danger is. In Chapter 3 we talk more about why the fear persists even when the danger is past, and in Chapter 4 we discuss how treatment can help. For now, keep in mind that the intrusions are a sign that the trauma is "unfinished business," and moving on usually means making sense of the past to be able to put closure to it and live in the present.

Hyperarousal

After a traumatic event some survivors remain on alert in many situations. In fact, they may have a hard time relaxing anywhere. A survivor may not recognize that she's safe, so she constantly reacts to the environment as if the perceived danger were real. Our brains have a system for protecting us against danger, known as the "fight–flight response." Once a person's brain perceives a threat, it directs her to continue scanning the environment for signs of danger. This helps her be prepared next time around.

Hypervigilance

Most people who have experienced trauma settle down after a while and reclaim a sense of safety. Some trauma survivors, however, remain **hypervigilant**, or "on alert," especially in certain situations. They examine their surroundings carefully, scanning for anything that may pose a threat to them or their family. For example, whenever Jenny and Marcus went out to dinner, she noticed he had to sit where he could see everything. This way he could check out every person in the restaurant to determine whether anyone posed a threat. One of the reasons Tom had trouble driving after his car crash was that he tried to be aware of everything around him that moved. After having experienced trauma, Marcus and Tom didn't feel safe anywhere, so they were constantly looking around for any sign of danger. And when something sudden happens, the trauma survivor may react more strongly than those around her. One of the first things Juan noticed about Estelle after she was assaulted was that she was "**jumpy**" all the time. Whenever the phone rang, she would startle before realizing what it was.

Difficulty Concentrating

Many survivors of trauma often have **difficulty focusing their attention** on daily activities for extended periods of time. We all have limited mental resources and usually can only focus on one thing at a time. Trauma survivors often find their attention diverted by thoughts and feelings about the past or by scanning their environment for danger, leaving them little capacity to focus on what's in front of them. At dinner, Jenny could see that Marcus was watching everyone else in the restaurant. As a result, he wasn't listening to what she was saying. Joe found himself redirecting Tom when they were driving after Tom had missed turns he needed to take because he was so busy watching other cars. Some trauma survivors also experience difficulties with memory for day-to-day events, which can be severe enough to impair their functioning at work or during other activities.

Memory impairments can be one of the most disturbing complaints for trauma survivors, yet scientists do not fully understand why they occur. Research suggests that the brains of trauma survivors are functioning differently than they did before the trauma. Trauma survivors are so focused on reexperiencing the past and being on guard for present danger that they often don't notice new information if it isn't related to threat. As a result, new information that might be important to a work task is not processed and stored for later recall.

Anger Management Problems

Being "on alert" so much of the time can cause trauma survivors to feel irritable, even angry. Some survivors have **difficulty managing their anger**. The anger experienced by trauma survivors is generally more intense and longer lasting than the anger of those around them. Sometimes anger is related directly to memories or thoughts of the traumatic event. At other times anger is triggered by events in the present. On one occasion when Tom let Joe drive him somewhere, Joe was amazed at how Tom reacted when another driver got close to their car. He opened the window and started yelling, and Joe purposely slowed down to let the other car get away from them. His brother remained irritable and anxious for the rest of the ride and for about an hour after they got home. The anger experienced by the trauma survivor can be so intense that he may fear it. He may be afraid that allowing himself to feel the anger could cause him to lose control and do something he'll regret. Trauma survivors often manage anger by "stuffing it down" and withdrawing from the situation instead of expressing themselves. When Marcus thought about the suicide bombings he had witnessed, he became so enraged at the disregard for human life that he felt like killing someone. The anger scared him.

It's important to realize that in many cases the trauma survivor has good reasons to feel angry. He may have suffered an injustice or been violated, threatened, or harmed. Feeling anger is a natural reaction to such incidents. Nonetheless, anger that is disproportionately intense, pervasive, and all-encompassing can present serious problems for the trauma survivor and those around him, particularly if it leads to aggressive behavior.

Trouble Sleeping

What about when everything is quiet and there are no distractions? Even then, people who have been traumatized can have a hard time calming down. One of the most common problems survivors have after trauma is **difficulty sleeping**. There are many reasons for this:

- Besides the nightmares discussed earlier, some survivors feel *a need to stay on guard at night*. For Marcus, it was a struggle to close his eyes. While lying in bed, he listened for sounds of an intruder and felt uncomfortable whenever he started to let his guard down.
- Survivors also can *reexperience the trauma* in bed, particularly if that is where the trauma occurred. Jake, who had been molested by his uncle in his bed when he was a child, found that memories of the sexual abuse intruded whenever he lay down in bed.
- *Ruminating* also can interfere with sleep. Karen, who had been sexually assaulted by a military officer while in Afghanistan, often lay awake ruminating about her anger toward the perpetrator and the peo-

ple in the Army who she believed had covered for him. Similarly, Laura ruminated about how her problems were affecting her marriage.

When survivors of trauma do sleep, often their sleep is not restful. They may move around or talk while sleeping. Tom sometimes slept 6 hours a night but would still awaken feeling as if he hadn't slept a wink.

Hampering Activities and Relationships

Problems with arousal can persist and cause complications in everyday life that can affect you as well as the survivor. If the survivor in your life has trouble containing his anger, you may have started to avoid him because you're afraid of getting hurt. You might avoid going places with the survivor if he angers easily because you don't want to be embarrassed if he explodes in public. You also may be concerned that his anger will draw you into a fight or legal complications or, worse, that he might hurt someone. Wayne was one of Sergio's closest friends, but after Wayne came back from a stint with the Navy in Kuwait during the Gulf War, Sergio learned very quickly not to go out to bars with him. Wayne would drink too much and look for a fight, and Sergio had gotten punched on a few occasions and even arrested once after Wayne initiated an altercation.

If your loved one has difficulty sleeping, it can be more than just an inconvenience. Lucy had been scared enough when Ed's screams from his nightmares woke her out of a sound sleep. But then one night he rolled over onto her and started to choke her. She had to struggle to get away from him. That night did it for her. They never slept in the same bed again.

Avoidance Symptoms

Reexperiencing a trauma is very unpleasant, so it's no surprise that many survivors go to great lengths to avoid it.

Avoiding Associations with the Trauma

Many trauma survivors try to **avoid thoughts or emotions related to the traumatic event.** Whenever Estelle had a thought about the assault, she would get up and leave wherever she was and do something to distract herself. The drinking that Juan had become concerned about also was part of her effort to avoid. She thought about the attack less when she was intoxicated, and she wasn't as upset when the memory did enter her mind. Trauma survivors also may **avoid reminders of the traumatic event.** Jerry, who had been deployed to Iraq during the first Gulf War, was reminded of his own experiences every time he saw the news about the recent Iraq and Afghanistan conflicts. He started to avoid watching the news so that he would not be reminded of experiences that were difficult for him. Trauma survivors also may **avoid talking about** the trauma. After Freddie was injured on the job, his wife, Patricia, was very upset and wanted to make sure he was okay. But whenever she tried to ask him about the forklift accident and how he was recovering, he changed the subject or abruptly left the room. Some trauma survivors have **difficulty remembering important parts of the event**, which may be a form of avoidance. Sarah tried to push details of her assault, especially the worst parts, out of her mind. She could recall being knocked down and then being thrown out of a car but nothing in between.

Detachment from Others

In addition to actively avoiding thoughts, feelings, and reminders of the trauma, survivors may avoid in passive ways. For example, trauma survivors often **feel distant or detached from other people**, which may lead them to isolate themselves from others. Detachment can happen for various reasons:

- Trauma affects people profoundly, and often the trauma survivor has a sense of being somehow *different from others,* as if she doesn't fit in. Some survivors even believe that they're "damaged" and that this sets them apart from others. Jake, who had been sexually abused as a child, felt ashamed of what had happened to him. He believed that if people got to know him they would see how damaged he was. As a result, he kept a wall up between himself and others and had few close friends.
- Trauma survivors also may have *difficulty trusting and confiding* in others. They often feel that others cannot understand their experiences and their reactions to them. Isolating themselves from other

people tends to magnify the feelings of being disconnected. For example, after having been assaulted by two men, Estelle had difficulty trusting men in general. As a result, she avoided interacting with them whenever she could, which led her to feel more isolated. When people learned that Marcus had been in Iraq, they asked him questions that made him uncomfortable, so he started staying away from family gatherings, church functions, and other social events.

Loss of Enjoyment, Love, and Happiness

People who survive trauma also may **lose interest in things they used to enjoy**. This may be because they can no longer do those things without getting upset or anxious. Tom stopped going to baseball games with Joe because the crowds made him nervous. Loss of interest also can happen because trauma makes everyday life seem insignificant. Marcus used to spend Sunday afternoons with his friends either playing cards or watching football. After watching friends die in Iraq, and bonding with fellow soldiers who had saved his life and whose lives he had saved, these Sunday games just didn't seem that important anymore. For some trauma survivors, losing interest in things is a manifestation of feeling depressed, which we discuss further below.

This loss of positive emotions may affect many areas of the trauma survivor's life. Often, trauma survivors report **difficulty experiencing feelings like love or happiness**. They may not experience the same emotions about family or achievements as they did before the trauma. Sometimes, by trying to not feel the negative feelings, trauma survivors end up dampening down their positive feelings too. The emotional numbness may be apparent to others close to the trauma survivor, who might describe him as cold or uncaring.

Loss of Faith in the Future

The severity of the trauma, or the harm threatened or actually done, may leave the survivor with a feeling that life could end at any time, with little warning. She may come away from the experience with a **sense that her future will be cut short** and thus see no need to plan ahead. Trauma survivors may not attend to things like planning for retirement because they don't see themselves living that long. Tom doesn't see any point in painting his house or planting shrubs and small trees anymore. Why bother? He probably won't be around to see them grow.

Getting Stuck

Avoidance can cause problems in important areas of functioning. Abruptly leaving various situations negatively affects how the trauma survivor is perceived by others. Passive avoidance, such as detachment and numbing, can lead to disruptions in the survivor's important relationships and diminished support from others, contributing to depression. Lack of participation in enjoyable activities results in few sources of pleasure and reward and also can negatively affect mood.

If something is frightening, our natural inclination is to get away from it. For trauma survivors this urge to avoid is especially powerful. Unfortunately, avoidance also prevents the trauma survivor from learning that he is no longer in danger, as he was when the traumatic event occurred. Experts believe that avoidance keeps the other symptoms around because it limits opportunities to learn that the world can be safe. We talk more about this in Chapter 3.

Other Symptoms

So far, we have described the effects of trauma that can result in a diagnosis of PTSD. As we noted earlier, trauma can affect those who experience it in a variety of ways besides the symptoms of PTSD. Trauma can affect the survivor's emotions, behavior, and ability to cope with stress, all of which can interfere with the survivor living a healthy life.

Emotional Responses

Trauma survivors may experience a wide range of **emotions** in connection with the traumatic event. For example, after his war experiences, a soldier may feel **guilt** about something he did, guilt about not having done something that could have saved someone from serious injury or death, or "survivor" guilt because he walked away from an explosion unharmed when another soldier was killed. Injured service members sometimes feel guilty about not being able to stay in the war zone to help friends who are still there. Tom felt **guilt** after his car accident. He kept racking his brain trying to figure out why he came away from the accident without any injuries while the other driver spent 6 months in the hospital.

Victims of trauma also may feel **ashamed** due to what happened to them. They sometimes believe that the traumatic event happened because of something wrong with them, or the trauma "tainted" or "soiled" them in some way. Estelle felt ashamed because she believed that she must have done something to "lead on" the men who attacked her. Later, when she got home, she had a hard time telling Juan what had happened, in part because she feared he also would think she had participated. Sometimes trauma survivors feel ashamed because of how the trauma has affected them. Nadim had always prided himself on being hard-working and healthy. After he was mugged at gunpoint and pistol-whipped, he recovered physically but continued to have nightmares and intense fear when he was outside at night. He thought this meant he was weak, and he felt ashamed of his reactions. As a result, Nadim did not tell his wife, Wanda, what he was experiencing. In this way, shame can make it difficult for a traumatized person to get support from people in his life.

Many traumatic events involve some sort of loss. This can be loss of another person, loss of a physical function due to injury, or loss of a part of one's life. **Grief** is a natural response to loss. Avoiding thinking about the traumatic event can interfere with healthy grieving. Avoidance prevents the traumatized person from acknowledging and accepting the loss. Rather than resolving his grief, he remains stuck in it. Whenever he thinks about the trauma or is reminded of it, he feels intense sadness. After a fellow police officer was killed in the line of duty, Pedro tried to focus on his job and worked hard to find the men responsible. But whenever he saw TV programs or movies about police officers he started crying and then would leave the room to "get control of myself." By cutting off his sadness whenever he felt it, Pedro prevented himself from completing the normal grieving process.

Depression

Another very common experience of people who have been traumatized is **depression**. More than half of people who have PTSD also are clinically depressed. When we use that word, we do not mean just the emotion of feeling sad or blue, which as we have already discussed is a common aftereffect of trauma. Rather, depression is an ongoing state of intense sadness accompanied by low energy, loss of interest in things, low motivation, restlessness, changes in appetite or weight, trouble concentrating, poor sleep, and thoughts of guilt or worthlessness. **Thoughts about death or dying** are common among people who have been traumatized, especially those who are depressed. As noted above, some people who have been traumatized narrowly escaped death. As a result they frequently think about how close to death they are. They also may feel so helpless and frustrated about their symptoms that death seems like it would be a relief.

Suicidality and Self-Harm

Trauma survivors are at risk for suicidal thoughts and behaviors. There can be many reasons for this. Often the emotional reactions such as shame, guilt, anger, grief, and depression become too painful, and the survivor sees suicide as a way out. Sometimes circumstances of the traumatic event make life seem less meaningful or substantially diminish the survivor's self-worth. Occasionally, suicidal thoughts can lead to suicide attempts. The success of a suicide attempt usually hinges on the lethality of the means chosen by the trauma survivor. For example, a suicide attempt that involves use of a gun or jumping off a 20-story building is far more likely to end in death than one that involves taking pills or cutting one's wrists. Some survivors may engage in suicidal "gestures" in which they aim to draw attention to the degree of their suffering without really intending to end their lives. Regardless of the underlying cause, any expression of suicidal thoughts and/or suicidal behaviors is a strong sign that the survivor would benefit from the assistance of a mental health professional. If your loved one has expressed suicidal thoughts or engaged in troublesome behaviors, you should take these statements seriously. Don't try to handle the situation on your own; encourage your loved one to seek professional help, and even offer to accompany him to the appointment.

Sometimes people with a history of trauma hurt themselves without wanting to kill themselves. Examples of this may include cutting, scratching, or burning themselves. Although the causes of such behavior are complex and not well understood, there are several possible motives for deliberate self-harm. As we discussed above, trauma survivors often feel intensely uncomfortable emotions, such as fear, guilt, anger, shame, and sadness. Sometimes they may inflict physical pain to distract themselves from these emotions. Conversely, some trauma survivors hurt themselves because they feel numb. They inflict pain upon themselves so that they can feel something, anything, other than numbness. In some cases, trauma survivors cause injury to themselves as a means of punishing themselves for things they did during the traumatic event.

Dissociation

Some survivors of trauma react to stress by "checking out." During the traumatic event they may have felt so overwhelmed that they mentally detached themselves from the situation, perhaps by going somewhere else in their imagination or by simply focusing on a sound, image, or other sensation. After the trauma, they continue to check out when faced with uncomfortable situations. To others, they may seem "spacey" or like they are somewhere else in their mind. In extreme instances, these individuals may lose blocks of time when their focus of attention is somewhere other than in the present. This kind of disconnection, termed "dissociation," is not in itself dangerous, but, as you can imagine, it can cause significant problems in daily life.

Poorly Developed Life Skills

Some people who experience trauma early in life, such as survivors of child abuse, are affected in ways that go beyond the effects of the trauma discussed so far. When trauma occurs during critical years of social and emotional development, the experiences and the context in which they occur can **interfere with development of important life skills**. This can include skills for knowing how to manage one's emotions and respond to them in ways that are helpful and constructive, as well as skills for interacting with others that enable a person to have rewarding and healthy relationships. Individuals who lack these important life skills enter adulthood unprepared to cope with many of life's challenges. They tend to be moody and to respond to painful emotions in impulsive and sometimes destructive ways. Their relationships tend to be unstable and unhealthy.

Substance Abuse

Some survivors of trauma turn to alcohol and drugs to help them cope with their symptoms. In moderation, this may not be a problem. But when use of substances causes more trouble than it resolves, it is considered **substance abuse**. A person who feels helpless in dealing with persistent grief or anger may resort to drugs like cocaine or heroin to change his mood. Or, as in Estelle's case, a trauma survivor may abuse alcohol in an effort to escape from relentless trauma memories and emotions or to get needed sleep. Substances can give trauma survivors a reprieve from their symptoms and a temporary sense of control over their lives. Unfortunately, the effects of substance use are short lived. The trauma survivor who relies on substances to manage her symptoms may feel less in control over the long term.

Reckless Behavior

Some trauma survivors engage in **reckless or thrill-seeking behavior**. In some cases, survivors miss the excitement or "adrenaline rush" they experienced during the trauma. After Wayne returned from his deployment, the everyday world just was not exciting enough, so he started driving fast, drinking a lot, and starting fights. For other trauma survivors, dangerous behavior may represent an effort to restore a sense of control. Marcy, who had been raped by a man she met in a bar, returned to the same bar several times, drinking and flirting with disreputable men to try to prove that she could conquer the situation.

Possibilities Now and in the Future

No two trauma survivors are affected by their experiences in the same way. At this time, we cannot predict how traumatic events will affect those who survive them. We do know, however, that your loved one's reactions after trauma may be influenced by various aspects of who he is. First, his biological vulnerability (his inherited tendency to be emotionally reactive) will help to determine his reactions. Second, his life experiences before the trauma play an important role. Through these experiences he learned what to expect from the world and how to cope with stress and unpleasant emotions. Finally, his reactions are affected by the connection he feels to other people. People with lots of support from family and friends tend to fare better after major life stressors.

It is important to note that not all people who suffer in the aftermath of trauma will display every symptom we've described. For example, Tom feels as though his life can be cut short at any time, but Estelle does not. Although Estelle drinks more than is healthy to cope with her symptoms, Marcus does not. So it would not be unusual if you recognize in your loved one only some of the problems described. She likely will not experience all of them. Also, the number of symptoms she experiences does not necessarily reflect the severity of her distress or how much the symptoms affect her daily life. For example, one person may have many of the effects described in this chapter and still be able to hold a job and meet personal responsibilities, whereas another might have only a handful of the symptoms that are so severe that he can't leave the house.

We've described the effects of trauma, so you may be wondering, "Okay, I understand some of the things I am seeing in my loved one, but what's going to happen now?" In Chapter 3, we talk about how these reactions to trauma interact with one another, how the effects of trauma change over time, and what can make the unwanted reactions last longer.

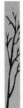

THREE

Why Is Your Loved One Stuck in the Past?

Kelly sometimes couldn't believe how good things were. When Steve first got back from Iraq, he was a mess. He would spring out of bed at random times during the night, breathing hard and sweating, for no reason at all. He would abruptly leave stores or restaurants and hardly ever seemed to open up to her about anything. But things slowly got better. After a month, he could sit through a meal in their favorite restaurant. After 3 months, he was sleeping through the night. Some things never quite went away. He still cried whenever he heard the national anthem, and she could see his eyes dart around whenever they entered a room. But these things really didn't make much of a difference in their daily lives.

Greg had thought Jeanette was fine after the mugging. She seemed to want to go right back out and get back to her regular routine. But after a couple of months, he recognized that she wasn't fine, not at all. It seemed to him that she was struggling to hold things together, and the more time went on, the more things seemed to fall apart. She started leaving work early because of anxiety attacks, and once she was in the house, she was in for the night. Greg didn't know what to think. Weren't things supposed to get better over time?

Andy was pleased with how fast they rebuilt after the tornado. But sometimes Lilly scared him a little bit. She had insisted on making

the house really secure, and he didn't know whether she was being
smart or paranoid. Only two walls of the house had windows, and
they had spent a fair amount more than the insurance company
gave them to reinforce parts of the building. The tornado had been
a sort of freak occurrence, and they weren't really in a high-risk area
for weather events. Was it just a case of better safe than sorry?

The effects of trauma can change greatly over time. Right after
the traumatic event, it is likely that your loved one will experience at
least some of the effects we discussed in Chapter 2. Several months
after the trauma, however, most survivors will have returned to life as
usual. Any remaining effects of the trauma probably will not cause significant problems. For a minority of trauma survivors, however, posttraumatic reactions can persist, despite being in a safe and supportive
situation. These survivors often can benefit from the numerous treatments available for the negative effects of trauma. In this chapter we
talk more about how you can expect the effects of trauma to change
over time and why some survivors' symptoms fade away while others'
problems persist.

How Will Things Change over Time?

In the immediate aftermath of a traumatic event, most of the people
who experienced it will be affected by it in some way. For example,
if we went into Andy and Lilly's town soon after the tornado hit and
asked the residents how they were doing, most would report that they
were not doing well at all. A majority of people would report problems
like poor sleep, nightmares, troublesome memories of the tornado, irritability, and trouble concentrating. And if you consider how frightening and destructive a severe tornado can be, this makes sense. It would
be surprising if the large majority of citizens did *not* experience distress
in the days and weeks right after the event.

For most people, the effects of trauma subside over time. If we
returned to Andy and Lilly's town 6 months or a year later, most residents would report that they were doing all right. The nightmares
would have stopped, the memories would have become less intrusive,
and they would be feeling calmer during the day and sleeping better at
night. Recovery is the natural course after a trauma, and most people

will return to normal life. A small percentage of the town's residents, however, would continue to experience the symptoms that started after the tornado. They may have lessened in frequency or intensity, or they might have worsened, but they would still be severe enough to interfere with daily life.

Delayed Symptoms

In some cases, the survivor may appear fine right after the trauma but then develop symptoms months or even years after the event occurred. Frank had gotten a job 3 weeks after he left Vietnam in 1969. He then worked for over 40 years, often putting in long hours and sometimes taking a second job above his work as a carpenter. When he finally retired and wasn't busy all the time, he gradually began thinking more and more about Vietnam. Then he started having nightmares. Jane was physically abused by her father as a child. She learned to cope by "boxing up" her feelings and "hiding them in the closet" while trudging forward with her life. It wasn't until her own children were toddlers that she was bothered by thoughts of the abuse, wondering, "How could anyone treat a child that way?"

It is not clear why some survivors develop symptoms immediately after the event whereas others develop them after a delay. As with Frank and Jane, in many cases of delayed onset, shifting life circumstances bring trauma memories to the forefront. Those memories demand the survivor's attention in a way that he can no longer ignore. This can be particularly perplexing for the trauma survivor and loved ones. Loved ones may have known about the event but thought it was all "water under the bridge." After all, it happened in the past, *and* it hadn't been an issue for so long. If your loved one began to have problems after a period of apparently normal functioning following the trauma, the changes in her can be unexpected, unwelcome disruptions to the status quo. You and the survivor probably would like things to go back to the way they were.

Memory Loss

In rare instances, the survivor may have had little or no memory of the event. As a result, she may not have been bothered by memories or avoidance of reminders during the delay period. Larissa had dissociated when her cousin was molesting her. Forty years later she saw a photo of the extended family at a picnic in which her cousin had posed with his arm around her. The memories suddenly flooded back, and she was horrified and overcome with shame. This was extremely confusing for her husband, Carlos, who had always noticed that she got a little "spaced out" when they were intimate but otherwise was not aware that anything bad had ever happened to her.

It should be noted that complete loss of memory of a traumatic event is exceedingly rare. In most instances the person realizes that at some level she had always been aware that the event had occurred. For the 40 years prior to seeing the picture, Larissa had experienced little distress about the abuse. Yet she had always felt repulsed by her cousin and avoided contact with him. Also, she knew that the numb feelings that came over her when she was intimate with Carlos were not "normal." When she thought about it, she realized that she had previously had "flashes" of her cousin touching her inappropriately when she was with her husband, which had led her to "numb out." Often, memories of traumatic events return when the situation and circumstances of the person's life make it safe to focus on them. In Larissa's case, her cousin had died that year, so she no longer felt as threatened by him.

The Controversy over Recovered Memory

The issue of "recovery" of trauma memories after a period of complete memory loss is a matter of considerable debate within the scientific community. Memory is vulnerable to suggestion and other outside influences. Sometimes a person can become convinced that a memory reflects actual events and feel intense distress about the recalled events, even when the events did not actually happen. In many cases of "recovered memory" that have led to accusations and criminal prosecutions of perpetrators, the victims later recanted. In some instances, memories of previously unrecalled traumatic events were found to have been introduced during a course of psychotherapy. A well-meaning therapist may have wrongly believed that certain patterns of symptoms were indicative of a history of childhood sexual abuse, leading the therapist to suggest this history to the patient.

Complete amnesia followed by recall can be particularly confusing for family and friends. It can help to support and validate your loved one, yet be cautious about the possible harm that can come from "false" memories. If you suspect that your loved one might have developed false memories, encourage him to proceed cautiously and to seek additional expert opinions.

Posttraumatic Stress Disorder

Posttraumatic stress disorder, or PTSD, is a specific disorder characterized by a combination of reexperiencing, avoidance, and hyperarousal symptoms that lasts for at least a month and interferes with the survivor's life. As noted earlier, most people believe that PTSD is a common consequence of trauma. In reality, it is not. Most who experience trauma do not develop symptoms that are persistent, pervasive, or disturbing enough to qualify as PTSD. In fact, 80 to 90% of trauma survivors will recover from the event. This does not mean that they are unaffected by the trauma. But distress is short-lived for most, and they resume their lives with minimal interference.

Some trauma survivors, however, experience persistent symptoms severe and disturbing enough to be diagnosed as PTSD. Individuals with PTSD often find it difficult to go back to functioning the way they did before the trauma. They may have trouble focusing at work, getting along with family and friends, and keeping up their usual activities—even things that they really used to enjoy. PTSD that persists untreated for many years can wear on the person. Eventually, those who suffer from the disorder may experience the deterioration in health that often is a long-term effect of high levels of stress.

The likelihood of developing PTSD varies for different kinds of traumatic events. For example, only about 4% of people who survive natural disasters will develop PTSD, whereas the rate for victims of child sexual abuse may be around 40% (Widom, 1999). **It is important to realize that some trauma survivors may experience symptoms that don't satisfy the requirements for a diagnosis of PTSD but still cause problems in their daily lives.** Recent research suggests that even "subthreshold" PTSD symptoms can have significant effects on long-term well-being that might be helped by treatment. For example, after the bus accident, Roxanne had strong physical reactions to seeing other accidents, and she had occasional nightmares. She also was highly watchful whenever she was in a moving vehicle, and she was easily startled. She avoided driving near the site of her accident and didn't like being a passenger in a car. Yet she didn't experience any loss of interest in her activities or the emotional detachment or numbing that many trauma survivors with full-blown PTSD experience.

Why Does the Trauma Continue to Cause Distress?

As explained in Chapter 2, avoidance is one of the three core symptoms of PTSD. Experts believe that avoiding people, places, and events that remind them of the trauma or that bring up thoughts and emotions associated with it prevents survivors from learning that the world is generally a safe place to be. Without this realization, they remain stuck in posttraumatic stress. Understanding this process can help you grasp what your loved one is going through and how you might encourage him to move forward.

Avoidance Interferes with Processing the Trauma

Research has begun to shed light on the reasons posttraumatic reactions continue for some individuals. Most experts on the effects of trauma agree that making sense of, or "processing," the trauma is an important part of recovery. A survivor whose processing of the trauma is interrupted may be more likely to experience sustained distress.

As we go about our lives, our minds are continually processing events that we experience. Our brains have a strong inclination to organize and catalog all the information we take in so that we can easily access it later. To do this, we have to think about what we experience and try to understand it. That way we can connect it with what we already know and access it later to help inform our decisions. *Processing* is the term used to describe that system of making sense of, organizing, and storing all of our experiences.

Think about what happens after you watch a movie with a lot of plot twists. You may find yourself going over the plot in your head several times, trying to make sense of the story. If you have a lingering question about some part of the film, it may continue to come into your mind and nag at you until you figure it out. After processing it you can file away your memory of the movie and turn to other matters without finding yourself distracted by it. Similar processing occurs after stressful events. Think about a stressful event from which you've recovered. Chances are that after it happened, you thought about it for a while, trying to make sense of it. You probably told other people your story, which also can help you process the experience. After a period of thinking and talking about it, you were able to leave it behind and focus on other things.

But what if you hadn't processed the event, either because other events interfered with processing or because, for various reasons, you didn't allow yourself to think about what happened? When Aaron was in Afghanistan, daily life was dangerous and he had to focus on survival. After the mission, during which his best buddy was killed, he couldn't afford to take time to process what had happened. He had to keep moving forward and focusing on keeping himself and others safe. The situation was similar for Grace, a survivor of domestic violence. After her husband, Luke, threatened her with a gun, Grace took her children and fled. For months she was on the run, moving from one safe house to another, staying on guard for signs of Luke and taking care of her children. She had no time to think about how frightened she had been when he threatened her or her feelings about their relationship.

Sometimes people avoid thinking about what happened because the memory brings up feelings that they feel unable to cope with. The event may have been so horrific or frightening that they dread feeling the fear or horror that comes up when they recall it. It's not uncommon for survivors to go to great lengths to avoid recalling memories of the events so they can avoid the feelings they had at the time. While a missionary worker in Africa, Nancy spent 4 months helping to dig wells before her entire group of 11 missionaries was captured by militants. While they were held hostage for several weeks, she witnessed several of her coworkers tortured, and two of them were beheaded in front of the group. Nancy was horrified by what she saw and felt terrified that she might be next in line to be killed in this way. After the group's release was negotiated, Nancy could not bear to recall the experience because she did not want to feel the horror, terror, and grief that the memories brought back. Nancy worked hard to stay away from the memories and images. As a result, she never really gave herself the opportunity to make sense of what happened to her. The memories and images were never filed away in her memory, and she couldn't feel safe back in her hometown.

Sometimes trauma survivors avoid thinking about the memories because they want to avoid "secondary" emotions that they experienced during or after the event. For example, Paul reported that when he was a guard in Iraq he was ordered to shoot a child who was carrying explosives. He was terrified that if the child came closer and detonated the explosives he and many others nearby would be killed, so he fired. Despite his sergeant's praise of him for having acted decisively to save many lives, Paul felt tremendous guilt, so he simply put it out of his mind. Similarly, Tess felt ashamed because she was sexually assaulted in a fraternity house at her college. She thought that because she was dressed in a short skirt and had been drinking and dancing with one of the assailants at the party, she had invited the assault. As a result, she didn't tell anyone what had happened or report it to the police. She didn't like how the shame felt, so she refused to allow herself to think about the assault.

In Chapter 2, we talked about how in some instances a person might disconnect from the traumatic event as it is happening, a process known as *dissociation*. This was the case when Henry, an experienced firefighter, was trapped by falling debris while attempting to rescue a victim from a collapsed building. At first he was panicked, but after a while he "zoned out" and went somewhere else in his mind. When Jeanette was held up at knifepoint, she responded "like a robot" and felt disconnected from the experience. Jessie was molested by her grandfather on many occasions when he was babysitting her between ages 5 and 7. She learned to escape the pain by pretending she was in a fantasy land with her favorite nanny. Years later, she had little memory of the actual events, quite likely because she was not mentally "there" when they happened.

Dissociation is considered a form of passive avoidance. It is a way of distancing oneself from the painful or frightening aspects of an experience when physical escape is not possible. A person who dissociates during an event is more likely to develop PTSD later. Some trauma survivors practice dissociating so often that it becomes a habitual way of coping. They come to rely on dissociation to deal with memories and unpleasant feelings associated with the trauma long after the actual event is over.

When a trauma survivor fails to process an event during or after the experience, the trauma memory remains "unfinished business." The survivor's mind will continue efforts to process the memory either at night in his dreams or when it is brought up by a reminder of the event while he is awake. Once the memory enters consciousness, it brings with it all the sensations, feelings, and meanings that the person associates with the event. When Aaron first got back from Afghanistan, he was busy settling back into life at home. But after a few months he had more time to think, so memories of that awful day when the mission went wrong started to come into his mind. At first he was overcome by feelings of grief, so he tried everything he could to stop himself from thinking about it. But his wife, Julie, realized something was bothering him and gently encouraged him to share the story with her. Initially he was reluctant because he didn't want to burden her with the horror that he had experienced. But after a while he realized that not sharing with her had put up a wall between them. Although sharing the story with Julie was extremely painful for Aaron, and difficult for her, it proved to be an important first step in moving on with his life. Subsequently, Aaron reconnected with some of the guys who were with him in Afghanistan and they talked more about what had happened. Disclosing his experiences to his wife helped him begin to process his experience and started him on a path to healing. Talking about that day in Afghanistan with Julie also had the benefit of increasing intimacy in their relationship.

Paul, on the other hand, could not bring himself to tell his wife that he had killed a child. He felt so ashamed of this fact that he refused to tell anyone or even let himself think about the incident. For example, when he saw a child on TV who reminded him of the child he had shot, he quickly changed the channel. He did everything he could to put it out of his mind, even if his behavior irked others around him. As time went on, Paul continued to avoid thinking about the event, but the more he did so, the more it seemed to surface in his daily life. Kids everywhere started to look like the one he had shot, so soon he was avoiding being anywhere where he might encounter children. Some days the shame was so intense that he didn't even want to be around people at all. It was like a black cloud hovering over him, and he just wanted to hide. When his wife questioned his behavior, he became terse with her and withdrew. Soon he was dreaming about the trauma, too. There seemed to be no escaping it. The harder he tried to put it out of his mind, the more it would pop up. Paul's avoidance of the memory had become an impediment to processing it, and as a result his mind would not let it go.

Perhaps the most difficult thing for survivors and their loved ones to understand about trauma is that the harder the survivor tries not to think about the event, the more often he thinks about it. This seems like a paradox. Shouldn't Paul's efforts to keep the trauma out of his mind lead to his thinking about it less? To understand this, take a second to imagine what Paul's day would be like. He would wake up and go about his day trying to stay away from everything in the world around him that might remind him of shooting that child. If he stayed home, he would think about what TV shows he could watch that would not have children in them. If he had to leave the house, he would work hard to stay away from any places that might have children in them. Even if Paul is completely successful and manages to stay away from all reminders of children, his brain, on some level, always knows that he is working to avoid children so that he won't be reminded of the trauma. Even when he is trying not to think about it, his mind is occupied with it the whole time.

Avoidance Interferes with Reduction of Fear

In addition to interfering with processing the trauma memory, avoidance is now understood to play a major role in perpetuating posttraumatic fear reactions. Let's consider how this works. During the traumatic event the survivor learns to associate aspects of the situation with danger. This is important for guiding future decisions about safety. So it happens automatically, even without deliberate efforts. For soldiers in a war zone it is critical to recognize that certain situations signal danger, and recalling those danger signals will help to ensure safety should that situation arise again. Danger signals can include aspects of the environment (e.g., time of day, location, temperature, sounds, or smells) and features of the threat (e.g., size, shape, color, or physical characteristics). When Marcus and his troop suddenly took small-arms fire while on a patrol, his brain automatically recorded aspects of the situation (e.g., the desert, nighttime, hot) and the threat (e.g., what sort of weapon, where the shooting was coming from) and cataloged these cues as danger signals. Later, when he was patrolling the same area, recognizing the same cues in the environment alerted him to be on guard to protect himself. In the war zone, cataloging and then accessing threat information is crucial for survival.

The same cues, however, may not signal danger in a different environment, such as Marcus's neighborhood after he returns home. Most soldiers, once they return home, will learn over time that these cues no longer signal danger. The more they have contact with the cues in the new, safe environment, the less anxiety those cues will trigger. Some returning soldiers, however, will continue to perceive these cues to be signs of danger and respond accordingly. This occurs when the soldiers avoid any contact with the cues and, as a result, have no opportunity to learn that they are safe in the new environment. For example, children were a danger signal for Paul because in Iraq insurgents sometimes used children as human shields and to carry explosives. After his return, his continued avoidance of children prevented him from learning that children in his hometown are not dangerous, as they were in Iraq. Paul's wife, Amanda, knew nothing of the situation with children in Iraq, so she was mystified by his avoidance of public places. Once she started to realize it was because he was avoiding children, she was even more confused. "He is being ridiculous," she thought. "He must know that children can't hurt him."

Paul's wife didn't realize, however, that we cannot talk ourselves out of fear. The only way out of fear is to learn something new *by experience*. Let's look more closely at how this works. Once fear is learned, the fear center deep in the brain, known as the *amygdala*, responds automatically to important information about danger. The amygdala launches a program of protective action whenever danger signals are encountered. When the amygdala is activated, it is as if an alarm bell sounds in the brain: "Danger! Danger! Red alert!" Paul learned to associate children with serious danger, so his amygdala responded as it was programmed to. The amygdala is all about emotion. It doesn't listen to "logic," which is based in the cortex (the outer layer of the brain, which directs most of our thinking). The cortex might tell the amygdala, "Settle down—there's nothing to be afraid of now. Children here at home are not the same as children in Iraq." But the amygdala is like the man from Missouri. "Show me!" screams the amygdala. "Prove that it's safe!" So the cortex might say, "Okay, stand right here next to the child and see what happens." The amygdala hears this and panics. "You want me to do what??!!" it screeches, frantically searching for a way out of the room. "Just stick around, and you'll see that nothing bad will happen," says the cortex, in a calm and steady voice. The amygdala has one main job: to protect life at all costs. So the amygdala doesn't take chances—it "plays it safe." From the amygdala's standpoint, it's best to stay away from those kids. Its motto is "Better safe than sorry."

Why Avoidance Seems Like a Good Option

Not surprisingly, it's a lot easier to listen to the amygdala and get out of the situation than it is to ignore the brain's danger signals (racing heart, rapid breathing, and other elements of anxiety) and stay in the situation. But unless the trauma survivor does precisely that, and chooses to stay in the situation despite how frightened he feels, he will never have a chance to learn that what he has been avoiding is actually safe.

It's completely understandable that many people cope with trauma by avoiding thinking about the events. In fact, you may have become painfully aware of how the memories affect the trauma survivor in your life, and you may have tried to help her avoid things that upset her. You may have encouraged her to avoid the memories by saying things like "put it behind you," or "no need to think about the past," or "let bygones be bygones." Even though Paul's wife, Amanda, didn't understand why he was having so much difficulty since he came back, she was quick to protect him. If a family member asked Paul about his experiences in Iraq, she would immediately intercede on his behalf, saying, "It's best not to get into that" or "Let's not go there; it's not good for him." As a result of his own desire to avoid and his wife's support of this coping strategy, Paul passed up many opportunities to process his memories, so after a while avoidance became a deeply ingrained habit. This was okay in the beginning, but soon it became clear that Paul's distress about Iraq was not getting better, and his functioning in daily life was getting worse. Paul did little but mope around and bark at the kids, and most days he didn't even leave the house. Amanda felt at a loss to understand why her love and support were not enough to help him get back into life at home. Gradually she began to realize that Paul needed help, but she didn't know what to do—she didn't know what kind of help was out there or how to get Paul to seek it out.

Besides protecting the survivor from memories and conversations, you may have helped her avoid places or things that remind her of the trauma. Roxanne often drove several miles out of her way to avoid the site of the bus accident. Her husband, Mitch, was okay with this. In fact, he didn't like being reminded of that day either. So even when he was driving, he decided it was best to stay away from that corner, and he took the long way around. After several years, it was still their habit; they didn't even talk about it anymore. Neither of them thought of this avoidance as bad. On the contrary, they didn't like being reminded of the accident, so they both thought avoiding it was best for them.

Please understand that trying to avoid uncomfortable situations is a perfectly natural tendency. You and the trauma survivor are not wrong or bad if you've both been engaging in avoidance. After all, the safest way to deal with a threat is to escape from it. Unfortunately, the "threat" that the trauma survivor is trying to escape is with her all the time, in the form of memories, thoughts, and unpleasant emotions. And even though having memories and feeling emotions can make it seem to the survivor as if the trauma were happening again, in reality memories and emotions cannot hurt her. She is in no real danger. Avoidance prevents her from learning that memories cannot actually harm her, and it interferes with the survivor's learning that everyday situations are safe. It prevents her from processing her memories and moving forward with her life. As you begin to notice the detrimental long-term effects of avoidance, you may realize that these outweigh the short-term benefits it provides. Keep in mind that avoidance produces short-term gain for long-term pain!

Treatment

Despite all the difficulties caused by avoidance, the prospect of thinking about the trauma and returning to normal life can be overwhelming for the survivor. He may have no idea where to start, and he probably doesn't know how to process the trauma on his own. The effects of trauma can be so severe and life-changing that both survivors and loved ones may wonder whether life can go back to the way it was. If the survivor can't work, interact with others, or even leave the house, it may be hard to imagine symptoms improving or going away. After several months of watching his brother's world become smaller and smaller, Joe started to wonder whether Tom would ever return to the way he used to be.

This is where treatment can help. As recently as 20 years ago, little was known about the treatment of PTSD. Since that time, however, there have been tremendous advances in our understanding of the disorder and research has produced several effective treatments. These treatments can decrease or eliminate PTSD symptoms and help the trauma survivor get his life back on track.

What You Can Do

We talk more about treatment for the effects of trauma in Chapter 4. For now, we'll discuss how you can help the survivor overcome avoidance and reach out for help.

Helping Your Loved One Decide to Change

In the same way that it impedes processing the trauma and reducing fear, avoidance also can interfere with the process of getting help. Doug's roommate, Will, was concerned about having a diagnosis of PTSD in his medical record, because it might have consequences down the road. But he also was hesitant to talk to someone about the shooting because that would mean he would have to think about it, which he was not ready to do. Similarly, Estelle struggled with feelings of shame about what had happened to her. She was scared to talk about it because she thought she would be judged based on the fact that she had been sexually assaulted.

Many of the effects of trauma can make it difficult for your loved one to seek help. The pervasive and progressive effects of avoidance can make it hard for trauma survivors to leave their comfort zone. Difficulty trusting others can make it hard for trauma survivors to open up to treatment providers. First and foremost, seeking treatment involves a break in routine and an immediate risk. Finding and traveling to see a treatment provider can be a daunting prospect. Those who have been living under an assumption of danger often have difficulty imagining a life that is not dominated by fear. Estelle circumvented some of these difficulties by starting with a health care provider she already knew and trusted, and this worked well for her. She told her gynecologist, whom she had been seeing for more than 10 years, what had happened. Her gynecologist was very sympathetic and supportive, and she talked to Estelle about how assaults can affect women and how treatment can help. She gave Estelle the name of a colleague who specialized in treating victims of assault, and Estelle was glad that she had been able to get help from someone she knew. She was fortunate to have such a person in her life. Many trauma survivors start out by talking with their family doctors. Those who are unsure where to turn for help can start by consulting a counselor in an employee assistance program, occupational health clinic, or student counseling center, or a pastoral counselor.

People seek professional help when the strategies they have relied on to cope are not helping them meet their needs. After all, if the way your loved one has been coping was working well, there would be no need to change. At some point it becomes apparent that old tried-and-true methods that worked in the beginning—during or immediately after the traumatic events—are no longer contributing to a satisfying life. The old coping strategies may have helped your loved one survive a frightening experience and might even have helped him make the transition back to "life as usual." But there are costs to these ways of coping, and after a while the costs may outweigh the benefits. For some, avoidance may have become so ingrained that the trauma survivor and those around him may not even be aware of these patterns and their effects on daily life. In other cases, family and friends are very aware of the costs of avoidance in terms of its effects on social and family life, and they are hoping to see a change. But the trauma survivor may be reluctant or even unwilling to leave his comfort zone. If he is to seek help, the trauma survivor must eventually conclude that he has more to gain by seeking help than by continuing his efforts to cope on his own.

Often when trauma survivors start treatment, their loved ones don't know what to expect. Marion thought her father would go back to the way he was before he was deployed to Iraq. But even after working hard in therapy and dealing with his nightmares and daytime memories, Marcus remained a different person than he had been before his deployment. Roger's wife, Diane, thought he could probably accomplish more than learning to "manage" his symptoms. But he had been struggling for more than 40 years, ever since he returned from Vietnam. Realistically, how much could she really expect him to change?

An Exercise That Can Help

Many different factors can affect a complex decision like whether to continue avoiding or to change and seek treatment. Putting all the considerations in one place, on paper, enables you to take everything into account at once and try to make as informed a decision as you can. One way to accomplish this is through a structured analysis of the costs and benefits called decision (or pro–con) analysis. The form on page 62 is a very basic decision analysis worksheet that breaks down the consequences of two different options into the pros and cons for the short and long term. Estelle may feel better for the next month if she continues to avoid thinking about the rape. Seeking treatment, on the other hand, would mean she would probably have to talk about what happened, which would be uncomfortable for her. So in the short term, avoiding treatment is the less distressing option. But in the long term, nothing would change, and perhaps her world would get even smaller as avoidance continued to take parts of her life away.

You can start the pro–con analysis as an informal discussion with your loved one. Note the short-term benefits of not getting help and the longer-term costs of continuing PTSD symptoms for his life. For example, the day after Estelle decided not to go to a party her sister was throwing, she felt more depressed than usual. When Juan asked her, she said she felt bad about not being there to support her sister. Sensing that Estelle might be getting fed up with her life being run by avoidance, he asked her what else she missed. He was surprised to find that she was aware she had distanced herself from their friends and that this bothered her a lot. She also mentioned that she knew her withdrawal was affecting him. They talked about the short- and long-term effects of continuing to avoid, and Estelle seemed trapped between the protection of avoidance and the loss of her friends and family. Then Juan brought up the prospect of treatment. Estelle was terrified of disclosing the assault to someone she didn't know. But she could see that if she did, she might feel like she was in control of at least part of her life. Juan asked her what things might be like in a year, or 5 years, if she got help. Estelle was struck by the lack of real long-term drawbacks to treatment. If it worked, she could have her life back, and all the struggles might be a memory. It was this discussion that tilted Estelle's motivation toward getting help. (You can see her considerations in the pro–con analysis on page 62.)

As you work through a consideration of pros and cons with your loved one, be aware of your own reactions to the prospect of change and a return to how things used to be. It is important to consider that as much as you desperately want your loved one to get better, there might be a part of you that doesn't want to see her change at all. For example, Jessie's boyfriend, Alex, really wanted her to get better because he missed being intimate with her. On the other hand, before the PTSD, she used to be very social—more social than he liked to be. He actually *preferred* being homebodies the way they had been lately. Eva wanted Mark to get better, but she also realized that while he was in Afghanistan she had worn the pants in the family. She took charge of everything from finances to housekeeping, meal planning, and their social schedule. Since he came back from Afghanistan, he had never really seemed able to take much on again, and she just continued. She had grown used to making all the decisions and liked how she felt competent, in charge, and needed by the family. If Mark got better, Eva might have to learn to let go of some of the control she had and let him participate in decisions more. She wasn't sure she wanted that. If you find yourself resisting such changes in your loved one, ask yourself whether you're doing so to avoid something that makes you uncomfortable. Consider how this may affect your loved one and your relationship with him in the long term.

"I Want the Old Jim Back": Accepting Change

Juan often found himself thinking back to what Estelle had been like when they first met. He wanted things to be like they were back then and wondered whether Estelle would ever be the same again. Connie, whose husband, Jim, was horribly burned in an accident at work, felt like she was living with a different person from the man she had married 17 years ago. Most nights, as she was falling asleep, she would reminisce about their life before the accident and think to herself, "I want the old Jim back!" You may have thought something like this yourself since your loved one experienced trauma. It is common for the loved ones of trauma survivors to want things to go back to the way they were. You may have hoped that any changes due to trauma could be undone and your loved one could go back to the way she was before the trauma.

Unfortunately, what happened happened; the traumatic event cannot be undone. It is impossible to go back in time and change that fact. It also is not possible for your loved one *not* to be affected by trauma. We are all affected in large or small ways by the things we experience. A trauma, by definition, is an event that is outside the realm of everyday life, and involves intense, unpleasant emotions, so it

Decision (Pro–Con) Analysis of Whether to Get Help

	Short-term		Long-term	
	Pros	Cons	Pros	Cons
Continuing as I am				
Getting help				

From *When Someone You Love Suffers from Posttraumatic Stress* by Claudia Zayfert and Jason C. DeViva. Copyright 2011 by The Guilford Press.

Estelle's Decision (Pro–Con) Analysis of Whether to Get Help

		Short-term		Long-term	
		Pros	Cons	Pros	Cons
Continuing as I am		I don't have to think about it any more than necessary. I don't feel as anxious or as ashamed.	I'm too scared to do anything. I have dropped out of my sister's life. I don't see our friends anymore. I'm hurting Juan.	I can maybe keep protecting myself from bad feelings. I might get better on my own.	I probably won't get better.
Getting help		I can feel like I'm doing something, like I have some control.	I'll have to think about it and feel those feelings. I have to talk to someone and tell him what happened.	I might get my life back. I might see my sister and my friends more. I might be able to go out with Juan.	It might not work.

is likely to affect us. For example, after their daughter Tess was raped, Ian and Maggie thought she would be "messed up in the head" forever. They were skeptical when she told them she wanted to get help. But they drove her to the therapy sessions anyway, and Ian took her for ice cream afterward, just like he had when she was a child. After 6 months, they were thrilled to see that Tess was taking her life back. She was resuming many of the activities she used to enjoy, and she had even started dating again. She seemed happy. But she also had started volunteering at a domestic violence shelter and, whenever the topic of women being discriminated against came up, she became really angry. Maggie and Ian were scared when Tess called them from jail one day, asking to be bailed out. She had been at a protest opposing legislation limiting restraining orders against abusive partners. Police had arrested her and four other women for refusing to move off the steps of the state capitol. To their surprise their daughter, who had always been law-abiding, was excited about her experience and talking about becoming even more politically active.

Keep in mind that recovery from trauma does not mean returning to exactly how things were before the trauma. Processing the traumatic memories involves making sense of what happened and moving forward with that new information. Tess was no longer having symptoms related to the rape, and she was able to live her life without being restricted by avoidance. But she had learned from her experience that women face difficult struggles in society, and often their voices are not heard. She vowed to speak up to oppose victimization of women.

Too often we think of the changes caused by trauma as negative (like the symptoms we discussed in Chapter 2). You may be surprised to hear that trauma also can lead to positive changes in those who survive it (we talk more about this in Chapter 12). The main thing to realize is that trauma, like anything else a person might experience, will have lasting effects on the survivor in your life.

The Bottom Line: Be Willing to Help, but Accept Limits

As you come to understand the effects of trauma and recognize them in the trauma survivor in your life, we hope you'll stop blaming him (and yourself) for the problems you're both having. This does not mean that you should stop trying to change for the better or that you have to accept things as they are. It is critical that you take care of yourself and make sure your needs are met as your loved one struggles with the effects of trauma.

Be willing to provide whatever help the trauma survivor in your life is ready to accept. If she is motivated to change and would like your help, reading and rereading this book may help prepare you to assist her in treatment. If she asks for your help in choosing a therapist but wants to work on therapy homework alone, do what you can and accept her boundaries. If she would like you to spend time with her after her therapy sessions, then do your best to be there for her. If she tells you she doesn't want to talk about her therapy at all, wait for her to bring up the topic. Be ready for the survivor to ask you for help, but also realize that she may keep things from you that she's not comfortable talking about. If, on the other hand, the trauma survivor wants nothing to do with treatment, then unfortunately all the knowledge in the world won't help you help her. It can be a very difficult balancing act to encourage and support the trauma survivor in your life without pushing her too hard and driving her away from treatment. But, with practice, you can find that balance and provide the best support possible.

FOUR

Treatments That Can Help with PTSD and Other Problems

Diane wasn't sure this treatment thing was working out. In the beginning, Roger had no desire to go to the VA. When he finally caved in to her demands and went, he came back sad. He had run into other Vietnam veterans, and initially this had made him feel comfortable. But after they told him that he would be sick forever, that PTSD couldn't be cured, he became so disheartened that he didn't even schedule an appointment with a psychiatrist. Why bother? The other vets said the staff would only help him learn to "manage" his symptoms, which he was doing fine on his own.

Wanda was crushed. She had been so excited when Nadim told her that he looked up a therapist in the phone book. He had struggled so much since the assault, and she thought he might finally be able to get back to being his old self. But after three sessions, he stopped going and seemed even more distraught than he had been before. When she finally convinced him to tell her what happened, he said that he got really scared when the therapist started talking about "reexperiencing" the attack in therapy. Nadim had no idea why she would want him to do that, and she never really explained it. Did the therapist really "specialize" in treating PTSD? Or did she just say that? He looked so sad that Wanda didn't know what to say. After the big risk he took, he seemed terrified to try again.

Julie was really glad Aaron was getting help. Ever since he came back from Afghanistan he hadn't seemed like his old self. She knew there were some rough times over there, and that losing his best friend was a major blow. Even so, she thought he'd perk up after a few months back home, but he didn't—in fact he seemed to get more depressed as time went on. His brooding was really starting to worry her. His therapist had said that cognitive therapy might help him out of this funk, but she wasn't quite sure what this meant. Really bad stuff happened over there. Could Aaron really think his way to feeling better about war?

How Treatment Can Help

Trauma survivors who still have symptoms a year after the event likely will continue to experience them unless they receive treatment. If you're reading this book in the first weeks or months after your loved one was traumatized, then it's a good bet that she will recover with support from you and others in her life. If it's been months or even years since the trauma and she's still struggling with unpleasant memories, painful emotions, and avoidance, professional treatment may help.

Recall from Chapter 3 that recovery from trauma typically entails (1) processing the memory, which helps the survivor reevaluate the meaning of the event, and (2) learning that the old danger cues no longer signal danger in the new, safe environment. If your loved one is suffering from PTSD months or years after the traumatic experience, she didn't make the transition from expecting danger around every corner to assuming safety. Fear is the driving force behind most cases of PTSD, and therefore the lion's share of the work in treatment is aimed at helping the survivor learn to feel safe again. Along the way, the trauma survivor also may need to resolve other unpleasant emotions, such as guilt, shame, anger, and grief, which, in addition to being sources of distress in themselves, can interfere with processing trauma memories. Psychological treatment for PTSD therefore is usually about facing fears and focusing on unpleasant memories to process and resolve the distress they cause. Doing so will result in fewer nightmares, less daytime distress, less time spent "on guard," less of that "wound-up" feeling, and less irritability. Treatment can eventually lead to more involvement in relationships with others and resumption of life activities.

Medications provide another treatment option that many trauma survivors find helpful. However, people have varying attitudes about what kind of help they would like for PTSD. Some trauma survivors prefer to "just take a pill" and are not interested in "talking with a stranger" about deeply personal matters. Others are completely opposed to medications for various reasons, such as concern about side effects and risks, desire to solve problems through their own efforts, or a preference to do things "naturally." In many cases people opt to rely on both medication and therapy, although there is minimal research to guide planning of combined treatment. In our society medications are more commonly available than therapists trained to deliver effective treatments for PTSD. Therefore, medication often is the first form of help offered to people with PTSD, by either their primary care practitioner or a mental health specialist. Even for those who prefer talk therapy, medication can sometimes offer short-term improvement in sleep, mood, nightmares, or other symptoms so that a person can function better until he can do the work of therapy, which can be a longer process.

Therapy entails making a change in coping methods. Many who suffer from PTSD are, unfortunately, reluctant to alter their well-practiced avoidance strategies. The decision analysis in Chapter 3 can help: it often reveals that the costs of those avoidance strategies outweigh the benefits. If that's the case for your loved one, the good news is that, with the help of a knowledgeable and skilled therapist, she can achieve significant changes within several months. Although there are many different approaches to therapy, only certain methods have been shown to produce reliably good outcomes for individuals with PTSD. These treatments help trauma survivors change their coping methods and focus on resolving distress directly related to the trauma, thereby improving the quality of their lives. Across all of these therapies, 67% of patients who completed treatment no longer met criteria for PTSD at the end of treatment (Bradley, Greene, Russ, Dutra, & Westen, 2005). The following table summarizes available information from research studies of treatments for PTSD that reported the number of patients who completed treatment who were free of the PTSD diagnosis afterward. The treatments are discussed below, beginning with those with the most research support. We've listed the full references for the research summaries that inform this chapter at the end in case you want to read more about the studies behind these conclusions.

Success Rates for Various Types of PTSD Treatment	
Type of therapy	Percent of treatment completers free of PTSD diagnosis
Exposure therapy	40–100
Trauma-focused CBT (exposure + cognitive therapy*)	45–94
Eye movement desensitization and reprocessing	77–90
Stress management	50–58
Cognitive therapy	42
Relaxation training	22
Supportive and present-focused therapy	10–40
No therapy	0–20

*Includes "cognitive processing therapy"

Treatment and Types of Trauma

Research has found that, regardless of the treatment, survivors of combat trauma tend to show the least improvement and survivors of sexual assault fare best (Bradley et al., 2005). An additional point worthy of consideration is that child abuse may affect social and emotional development in ways that may make it difficult for child abuse survivors to participate constructively in trauma-focused cognitive-behavioral therapy (CBT). Some child abuse survivors can have trouble engaging in trauma-focused CBT and/or show problems dealing with emotions and sustaining healthy relationships. In such cases, treatment that includes emotion management skills may have a greater likelihood of success both for resolving PTSD and improving overall functioning.

Exposure Therapy

According to research over the last 30 years, the most effective treatments are various types of **cognitive-behavioral therapy**, or **CBT**. CBT helps a person learn new ways of acting and thinking that can reduce emotional distress. Exposure therapy, often called *prolonged exposure,* is a CBT method that helps people overcome many kinds of fears. Exposure therapy has been widely used for many years and is effective for helping people with various anxiety problems reduce their fear and return to normal functioning. Over the last 15 years numerous studies have shown that exposure therapy works extremely well for PTSD:

- Research to date has found that exposure therapy produces the most robust and enduring improvements in PTSD symptoms and therefore is considered the first-choice treatment for PTSD (Foa, Keane, Friedman, & Cohen, 2009; Powers, Halpern, Ferenschak, Gillihan, & Foa, 2010).
- A recent review of the research (Ponniah & Hollon, 2009) found that 40–100% of patients who completed exposure therapy no longer met the criteria for PTSD after treatment, compared with 0–20% who did not receive treatment. For the vast majority, the improvement was maintained for at least 6 months and even as long as 5 years later. This research also shows that exposure therapy reduces general anxiety and depression and improves overall functioning.
- Studies of exposure therapy suggest that the average patient who receives exposure alone or as part of a treatment package is likely to experience a greater improvement in PTSD symptoms than 86% of those who receive supportive counseling alone. At follow-up, those who receive exposure are likely to fare better in terms of their PTSD than 76% of those who receive only supportive counseling. In terms of the effect on depression and general anxiety, the average patient who receives exposure is likely to show more improvement than 79% of those who do not (Powers et al., 2010).

Melissa's story illustrates what happens during exposure therapy. One spring evening as Melissa was walking to the corner store, she passed her neighbor's German shepherd, Oscar. He had always been calm and friendly before, so she didn't think twice about approaching to greet him. But, for reasons still unknown, Oscar suddenly turned on her, and, snarling and snapping, he chased Melissa across the street. As she fled in terror she stumbled and fell, hitting her head on the sidewalk and landing in a flowerbed. Oscar bit her several times in the face and abdomen. She screamed, and with a passerby's help she was able to fend off Oscar and run to safety. She was quite shaken up, and soon an ambulance arrived and took her to the hospital. Her extensive bite wounds were cleaned and stitched up, and in the months that followed she underwent several surgeries to repair the scars.

Before this incident, Melissa was not particularly afraid of dogs, but now she was terrified of them. At first she was just on the lookout for dogs that resembled Oscar. But over time the more she avoided situations where she thought there *could be* a dog like Oscar, the more her fear mushroomed, and eventually she feared all dogs. She completely avoided the street where Oscar lived, even though after the attack he had been put down and no longer was a threat to her. Also, although she wasn't fully aware of why, she found that she felt uncomfortable around flowers—one whiff of the bouquet her boyfriend brought her for Valentine's Day and she broke into a cold sweat with her heart pounding. Sheer terror overcame her. She waited until the next day to throw the flowers away, but all evening she had a knot in her stomach, and that night she had dreams of being chased by packs of barking, snarling dogs. Dreams like this were a regular occurrence, and many mornings she awoke feeling exhausted, dreading the day at work. It took all her energy to push aside the memories and focus on her job. Melissa confided in her doctor and she referred her to a psychologist who diagnosed her with PTSD.

The goal of exposure therapy is to help the trauma survivor overcome her fears. As the first step in therapy, Melissa and her therapist identified categories of things that she feared (her danger signals). Dogs, flowers, and the streets around Oscar's house all were fear cues for her. For each they came up with a list of variations of that category of cues and then made a plan for her to approach the feared cues systematically. For example, for the category of dogs, they started with pictures of dogs and then worked up to actual dogs, beginning with friendly puppies. Later they also worked on her fear of flowers and of walking on Oscar's street. This kind of exposure, in which the person learns that the fear cues—objects, situations, activities, people, or even colors or smells—no longer signal danger, is called **in vivo** exposure (in Latin, *in vivo* means "in real life").

During *in vivo* exposure, the survivor's anxiety often increases when she first approaches the fear cue. But if she stays in the situation long enough, her anxiety usually will diminish, as she learns that she is safe. Exposure therapy entails many repetitions of prolonged exposure. For example, for her first week of practicing exposure therapy, Melissa and her therapist made a plan for her to look at a photo of a dog for 30 minutes each day. Monday she felt intensely afraid, and her amygdala was urging her to escape from the photo. She was so distressed that she started to feel doubtful about the therapy and was regretting her decision to seek help. But logically, she knew the photo couldn't hurt her, and she reminded herself that this was an opportunity to overcome her fear, so she stuck with it. By Saturday she was barely anxious, and she felt more confident that this process could help. She started to realize that her fear of dogs was not accurately signaling danger.

In addition to fearing cues around her, Melissa also felt as if she was haunted by frightening memories of the attack. She hated the feelings that the memories brought on—terror and complete powerlessness—so it's not surprising that she did her best to push these memories away. As a result, she had not processed the memories of the attack and continued to feel frightened of them. Exposure therapy for PTSD also includes a form of exposure, called **imaginal exposure**, that focuses on reducing fear of the memories that the trauma survivor avoids. In this part of the therapy, the trauma survivor describes her traumatic experience repeatedly for a prolonged period (usually 30–60 minutes). As with *in vivo* exposure, imaginal exposure is most effective when practiced regularly. The therapist typically provides an audio recording that the client uses to guide practice at home. Listening to the recording daily will facilitate processing of the memory and reduction of fear associated with it. Therapy typically entails several weeks or more of practice with different trauma memories, or different parts of a trauma memory.

Although the primary aim of exposure therapy is to reduce fears of thinking about what happened, processing the memory often also reduces other emotions, such as guilt, shame, or anger. This occurs because processing the memory allows the survivor to consider relevant aspects of the situation that she didn't consider when she avoided it and leads her to reinterpret what happened. In the 1993 film *Fearless*, Jeff Bridges, as Max Klein, the survivor of a plane crash, tries to help a fellow survivor, Carla Rodrigo (Rosie Perez), who struggles with guilt over losing her infant, who flew from her lap during the crash. Max resorts to a dramatic demonstration to help Carla process her thoughts about the crash. He gets Carla into the passenger seat of a car with a heavy toolbox in her lap and then crashes the car into a wall, essentially re-creating the plane crash. Carla's guilt is assuaged when, by reexperiencing the event, she comes to appreciate that the forces were such that she could not possibly have held on to her son. It is important to note that exposure therapy does not involve a real-life re-creation of the trauma, but very often, by reliving the experience in her mind, the trauma survivor becomes aware of important details and facts that alter her perception of responsibility and lessen feelings of guilt or shame.

To some trauma survivors and their families, exposure therapy can seem confusing or even cruel. When Roger explained exposure therapy to Diane, she nearly called the VA herself to protest. Didn't his therapist realize that those memories were what scared Roger the most? Why would he ask Roger to think about them for extended periods of time? The procedures of exposure are counterintuitive to the goal of reducing immediate distress, so understanding the rationale for exposure is critical for making an informed decision about participating in it. A skilled therapist will take time to ensure that the trauma survivor fully understands the reasons for exposure therapy and, because your support is essential, also will include family members in the preparation process.

If you're having trouble understanding how this treatment could be helpful when it makes the trauma survivor in your life do what he fears the most, remember that he's already thinking about the trauma. If the trauma never came to his mind, he would not have PTSD and probably would not be having as much difficulty as he is having now. It also can help to keep in mind that exposure therapy works. As with many healing processes, such as when going through physical therapy for an orthopedic injury, sometimes we have to endure some measure of increased distress to recover fully.

Virtual Reality Therapy

Virtual reality is a method of exposure therapy that helps the trauma survivor relive the traumatic event by immersing the survivor in animated scenes viewed through a special head-mounted computer display. It is typically delivered by a therapist. Virtual reality programs have been developed for survivors of the Iraq war (*Virtual Iraq*) and the 9/11 World Trade Center attack. This treatment may appeal to people who are comfortable with computers. Still in its infancy, the research so far suggests that it can be helpful, though it's unclear whether it is any better than usual "low-tech" exposure therapy. However, this therapy is not widely available as it requires special equipment.

Cognitive Therapy

As the table on page 69 shows, there is strong research support for cognitive therapy in the treatment of PTSD, especially when it also encourages changing behaviors and processing trauma memories, as in trauma-focused CBT. Cognitive therapy for PTSD focuses on how the traumatic experience affects a person's thoughts and beliefs. Trauma tends to change how the survivor thinks about himself, other people, and the world in general. A central premise of cognitive therapy is that the way we think affects the way we feel. PTSD is often associated with extreme negative views of oneself and of the world. For example, the trauma survivor may believe the world is very dangerous and people can't be trusted. The trauma survivor also may blame herself for what happened, as Tess did after her sexual assault, or feel ashamed of his actions, as did Paul after he shot the child who was carrying the explosive. Sometimes the negative beliefs about oneself can become so pervasive that they lead to depression. The individual may feel that she is worthless or that her life is meaningless. This was the case for Jessie, who was molested as a child. Her entire life Jessie believed that her grandfather had treated her badly because she was "no good." Aaron also had such thoughts after he returned from Afghanistan and had time to think about his best friend's death in the war. He wondered, "Why did it have to be him—why not me?" Although this bothered him for a while, he was able to find meaning in his life over time, with the support of his family. Sometimes, however, the survivor can become stuck in a downward spiral of negative thoughts and feelings that can be hard to break out of on his own. The goal of cognitive therapy is to help the trauma survivor learn to be aware of and modify unhelpful ways of thinking that contribute to distress. In cognitive therapy the trauma survivor is encouraged to examine the accuracy of thoughts and beliefs about himself and the world that may have been affected by traumatic experiences. Sometimes this is accomplished by talking through what happened. But very often thoughts can be so jumbled inside our heads, especially when it comes to emotionally charged topics, that it works best to write things down. Ultimately, cognitive therapy involves learning the skill of thinking in realistic and helpful ways. Practicing by organizing thoughts on paper strengthens this skill. As with exposure therapy, practicing these skills at home between sessions is important for treatment to succeed.

Trauma-related thinking is often biased and extreme. The trauma survivor will tend to overpredict the likelihood of bad things happening and think in all-or-nothing terms that usually don't fit with reality. Cognitive therapy helps the survivor learn to think in more balanced, realistic, and helpful ways—to appreciate the subtle shades of gray in the world, rather than seeing things as all black or white. For example, Rob was bothered a lot by an encounter in Kosovo, where he thought his commanding officer had put the unit in danger to look good. Thinking that a soldier in charge of other soldiers would put them in danger for no valid reason was devastating to Rob, who had believed very strongly in the bonds among soldiers. After that event, he had a hard time believing in anyone in authority. When he left the military, he went about life in the civilian world thinking that no one in authority could be trusted. Although it is true that some people in authority positions are untrustworthy, certainly there are many authority figures who can be trusted. The reality is that most people in authority probably fall somewhere in the middle. But for Rob, it was an all-or-nothing concept—authority meant that no trust could be given. This way of thinking was causing him problems in daily life, especially at work, because he didn't trust his boss.

Survivors of trauma often are struggling to make sense of horrific events. In doing so they sometimes draw overly simplistic conclusions about those events and ignore everything else they know about the world. Cognitive therapy can help the survivor look at all aspects of the situation in ways that incorporate all the facts. For example, Paul believed he was a "despicable person" because he had killed a child. After all, in his life before Iraq, wasn't a "baby-killer" the worst possible thing a person could be? Nothing in his prior life experience had prepared him for the no-win situation he encountered—a bomb strapped to a child. He knew the explosives were enough to take out his entire unit as well as many civilians nearby. His commander ordered them to shoot the child to save them all. Through cognitive therapy Paul was able to see that, although his actions were in conflict with some of his values, he had to understand them in the context of the war rather than in the context of his prior life. Doing so allowed him to soften his stance toward himself. Although he accepted that in most (in fact, nearly *all*) circumstances killing a child was certainly wrong, in the situation he faced it was the lesser of two evils and resulted in scores of lives being saved. Though he wasn't quite ready to see himself as a hero, he became less of a demon in his own eyes. Lightening the burden of shame about his actions enabled him to move forward in processing other memories of the war. Like Paul, many trauma survivors get stuck trying to apply black-and-white rules to the very complicated situations that often characterize trauma. A major aim of cognitive therapy is to help the trauma survivor find a way out of the quagmire by broadening his view of the situation.

Cognitive therapy also encourages the trauma survivor to ask how well his beliefs work for him in daily life. For example, when Marcus started therapy, he went about his life focused on his belief that "people are cruel." His therapist pointed out that, although indeed it is true that human beings *can be* cruel (verified by what Marcus witnessed in Iraq), Marcus's experiences from his deployment did not prove that *all* people are cruel. Furthermore, she noted that when Marcus focused his thoughts on this overgeneralization he avoided people, kept himself isolated, did not notice the good things that people did, and generally felt pretty sour. With his therapist's help he altered his thinking enough to be able to experiment with spending more time around people.

To survivors of trauma and those who have watched them suffer and struggle, cognitive therapy can sound like it's not enough. Upon hearing about the treatment many trauma survivors ask, "With all I'm going through, how would writing down my thoughts change anything?" It's important to remember that human beings are *always* thinking. We are always saying things to ourselves, and these self-statements can have a strong effect on how we feel and what we do. By changing how we think, cognitive therapy often leads to changes in what we do. Many forms of cognitive therapy deliberately emphasize changing behaviors as well. Some forms of cognitive therapy (e.g., cognitive processing therapy) strongly emphasize challenging beliefs within specific themes that tend to be affected by trauma (safety, trust, power, esteem, intimacy). Besides improving the symptoms of PTSD, cognitive therapy has been shown to be effective for many of the problems associated with posttraumatic stress, such as depression and substance abuse. There is some evidence that cognitive therapy may be particularly helpful in cases in which guilt and shame are the predominant emotions.

Combining Forms of CBT

PTSD is a complex and multifaceted problem, and no two cases are alike. The constellation of emotions and symptoms is influenced by the nature of the traumatic events and the characteristics of the individual who experiences them. Research has shown that both exposure therapy and cognitive therapy can be effective by themselves. In many instances, however, a therapist may deem that both are warranted and the specific amount of each will depend on the issues that arise in therapy. Therapies that combine cognitive therapy with some form of exposure to trauma memories (including "cognitive processing therapy") are listed in the table on page 69 under "Trauma-focused CBT."

In her therapy Estelle had courageously faced the memories of her assault through repeated and prolonged exposure. During the exposure, her therapist noticed statements she made about herself, such as "I should have known they were dangerous" and "Why did I freeze up and not move?" Although her anxiety lowered during the exposure and her PTSD improved to a degree, her guilt did not improve, and she continued to become upset when reminded of the assault. Her therapist decided to add cognitive therapy to her treatment plan. He helped Estelle evaluate the evidence for these thoughts. This helped Estelle realize that she had done nothing to cause the assault and that she froze because she could not possibly have fought off two men. It took a lot of work, but when Estelle changed her thinking, she felt less guilty and her PTSD resolved more completely. Conversely, Marcus's therapy started out with primarily cognitive interventions. Challenging Marcus's negative beliefs about the world resulted in Marcus feeling less depressed and being more engaged with his family. His nightmares and fear in daily life persisted, however, so his therapist suggested that he consider adding exposure therapy to his treatment plan.

Eye Movement Desensitization and Reprocessing

Eye movement desensitization and reprocessing, or EMDR, involves the trauma survivor talking through the traumatic event and alternate ways to think about it while her eyes follow a target that moves from side to side. Research on EMDR has shown that it can produce comparable improvements to the various forms of trauma-focused cognitive-behavioral therapy that include some form of exposure. EMDR might be more appropriate for civilians with a single trauma than for veterans (Albright & Thyer, 2010) and those with multiple traumatic experiences and/or childhood trauma (Schubert & Lee, 2009). Originally, it was theorized that the treatment was effective because the side-to-side eye movement re-created the eye movement that occurs while we dream, which allowed the brain to process the trauma memory. Later research showed that the eye movements, which were thought to be the main mechanism of treatment, were not essential. If some other physical activity was substituted for eye movements, the treatment was still effective. This research led some researchers to conclude that EMDR is a form of cognitive-behavioral therapy. EMDR can seem strange to some people who hear about it. If research has shown that its most distinctive feature, eye movements, is not necessary for EMDR to be effective, then why use it? For some patients with PTSD, the eye movements may make the treatment more appealing or tolerable than the more straightforward approach of exposure therapy. If your loved one seems to be interested in EMDR, keep in mind that, regardless of the findings about eye movements, EMDR has been shown to be an effective therapy for PTSD.

Stress Management Therapies

Stress inoculation therapy was not originally developed to treat PTSD, but several studies have shown that it can reduce PTSD symptoms better than no therapy at all, though it is not as effective as trauma-focused

CBT. Stress management is a form of cognitive-behavioral therapy aimed at teaching the survivor coping skills for managing anxiety and stress in daily life. The form of stress management therapy that has been used most frequently in studies of PTSD is called **stress inoculation training**. The developer of stress inoculation training, Donald Meichenbaum, suggested that, as with inoculation against a disease-causing germ, exposure to low levels of stress can develop our capacity to respond well to high levels of stress later on. The method entails teaching the survivor various stress management skills and then practicing the skills under low-level stress conditions, both in the survivor's imagination and in real-life situations. The skills can include a range of anxiety management strategies, such as relaxation skills, assertive communication skills, and coping self-statements that help to manage increasing levels of discomfort as a stressful situation progresses. Even though stress inoculation skills help a person to cope with daily stressors, they do not address the problematic issues that arise directly from the trauma, which may be why this treatment is less effective than trauma-focused CBT.

Present-Centered Therapies

Present-centered therapies typically include a combination of "supportive therapy" and problem-solving methods to help the client cope successfully with the stressors that emerge in daily life. Several studies have shown that therapy that focuses on helping the trauma survivor resolve current life problems can be beneficial for some groups of patients with PTSD. This is not surprising, since persons suffering from PTSD often are coping with many additional stressors, both related and unrelated to the traumatic event. For example, military personnel returning from deployment often are coping with myriad challenges in readjusting to life at home. They may face unemployment, marital stress or divorce, custody disputes, family disputes, and other difficulties settling back into civilian life. Often such problems compound post-traumatic stress and can make it difficult, if not overwhelming, to try to cope directly with the trauma in therapy. In many instances, treatment may need to focus on helping your loved one resolve these problems before he can address the difficulties stemming directly from the trauma. In addition, because many individuals with PTSD are socially isolated, there can be significant benefit from receiving social support in the therapy relationship. Such therapy also can be a vehicle for help-ing them reconnect with other sources of social support in their lives. As we've mentioned elsewhere, although the reasons are not entirely clear, social support is an important factor in healing from trauma.

Present-centered, supportive, and problem-solving therapies can benefit the individual as a whole, though not as effectively as trauma-focused CBT, and they can produce noticeable, albeit modest, effects on PTSD symptoms. Many individuals suffering from PTSD can benefit if they are not willing or ready to engage in trauma-focused treatments or do not have access to a therapist trained in those therapies. At the very least, they can improve social support and reduce stress caused by life problems, and they may reduce PTSD symptoms to an extent. They also can serve as an eventual segue into trauma-focused therapy for those who are not ready to do the work it entails.

Imagery Rehearsal Therapy

Another promising type of CBT that may help trauma survivors who suffer nightmares is **imagery rehearsal therapy**, or IRT. IRT was devel-oped for the treatment of chronic, disruptive nightmares and has been successful in reducing nightmares among trauma survivors. IRT is similar to exposure but focuses specifically on recurring disturbing dreams. First the trauma survivor writes down a recurring nightmare in as much detail as possible. Then she chooses one part of the dream to change (this change may alter the whole plot of the dream, or it might just change the ending) and rewrites the entire nightmare account with that change. Each night before going to bed, she reads the changed account and then uses a relaxation technique. The trauma survivor typically also learns cognitive-behavioral methods for improving sleep along with IRT. Research has shown that IRT is effective for decreasing nightmares and improving sleep, and can improve overall symptoms of posttraumatic stress in patients who suffer nightmares.

Other Therapies

Other forms of treatment for PTSD are not included in the table that appeared earlier in this chapter because there is very little research on them. The few studies available on these therapies suggest, however, that they might help some people. Among them are conjoint CBT (which aims to enhance communication and intimacy in the marital relationship while processing the trauma; see Chapter 11), hypnotherapy (which entails connecting patients to the reality of the trauma and reducing conditioned responses associated with it), and interpersonal psychotherapy (which focuses on improving close personal relationships), as well as trauma-focused group therapy for PTSD. Interpersonal psychotherapy may have particular utility with survivors of childhood abuse, sexual assault, and partner violence. Trauma-focused group therapy is widely used in veterans' hospitals, and research suggests that veterans can benefit from it, especially when it includes exposure (Ready et al., 2008). You and your loved one also may encounter therapists who apply existing psychotherapeutic approaches to posttraumatic symptoms, such as a trauma-focused psychodynamic therapy, which aims to decrease PTSD symptoms by resolving "intrapsychic conflicts" associated with the trauma. Some psychodynamic strategies may, in fact, resemble aspects of CBT, but because psychodynamic therapies have not been as easy to systematize and study, there is less evidence that they work. Nonetheless, they may be helpful to those who have been unable to engage in CBT or failed to benefit from it.

In general, we advise caution when pursuing treatments for PTSD that are not supported by reputable research studies. By its nature, trauma involves frightening or horrific memories and highly repugnant emotions, and everyone affected would prefer an easy way to make "it" and the horrible feelings associated with "it" go away, as quickly and as painlessly as possible. So we often seek out the easiest solutions and hope for almost magical outcomes. As a result, we may be drawn to treatment methods that purport to shield the survivor from distress, or alleviate suffering in remarkably quick and easy ways. In reality, nearly 25 years of research on PTSD has shown us that there is no easy solution to this complicated problem. We have therapies that work, but they can be hard for all involved because they entail working through painful memories and emotions to transform the meaning of the trauma from destructive to neutral or empowering. Be skeptical of any treatment that claims to bypass this process. Also, keep in mind that therapy should aim not only to reduce PTSD and related symptoms but also to promote positive transformation and personal growth, and these benefits are reaped only with effort.

Medication

Research shows that certain medications can be effective for treating posttraumatic symptoms (Raskind, 2009). In particular, more than half of the patients treated with the antidepressants known as **selective serotonin reuptake inhibitors** (SSRIs) will experience at least a 30% drop in their PTSD symptoms, which most researchers agree is a significant change for the better. Also, Murray Raskind and his colleagues at the Seattle VA have shown that **prazosin,** a drug originally used to lower blood pressure, can reduce veterans' nightmares by 50% and improve sleep.[1]

Generally, the effects of medication tend to be smaller than the effects of psychotherapy, but medications are nonetheless widely used for the treatment of PTSD (Penava, Otto, Pollack, & Rosenbaum, 1996). Medications have two main advantages. They require minimal effort, and they often can produce treatment effects more rapidly than other treatments. Medications also have two limitations. First, they can have side effects and risks that may be unacceptable for some trauma survivors. Second, medications help only while they are being taken, whereas psychotherapy effects tend to endure well beyond the therapy period.

Antidepressants

These caveats aside, a variety of medications that were originally used for other problems can be helpful to treat PTSD and its associated symptoms. The most commonly prescribed medications for posttraumatic symptoms are **antidepressants.** The SSRIs are the most commonly used medications for PTSD. Two, sertraline (typically marketed as Zoloft) and paroxetine (Paxil), are approved by the U.S. Food and Drug Administration for the treatment of PTSD. Other SSRIs, such as citalopram (Celexa), fluoxetine (Prozac), and escitalopram (Lexapro), also are commonly prescribed. Research has shown venlafaxine (a **serotonin–norepinephrine reuptake inhibitor,** or SNRI, marketed as Effexor) to be equal to SSRIs in efficacy with posttraumatic symptoms,

---

[1]Although the researchers have not found effects on overall PTSD, studies have not yet looked at prazosin taken during the day. Studies of prazosin for civilians with PTSD are ongoing.

and it also is a recommended treatment. Other types of antidepressants, such as **tricyclic antidepressants** and **monoamine oxidase inhibitors**, also are viable treatments and are usually considered when SSRIs and SNRIs are not tolerated or fail to help.

Antidepressants do, however, come with risk for side effects, some of more concern than others. SSRIs in particular have been associated with a high risk for sexual side effects, which in most instances consist of difficulty achieving erection and ejaculation for men and difficulty achieving orgasm for women, although reduction in libido also can occur. Although the sexual side effects sometimes can be mitigated by medication, they are among the most common reasons for discontinuing SSRIs. In addition, antidepressants can take between 2 and 8 weeks to take effect, and it can take months for some persons to achieve full remission of PTSD. Also, it is important to keep in mind that their effects typically last only as long as they are prescribed and taken. A reduction in symptoms achieved through use of medication may require continuation of that medication to be sustained. Finally, although the issue is somewhat controversial, some patients have reported withdrawal symptoms when they attempt to reduce or discontinue medications, even antidepressants.

It is unclear why antidepressant medications are helpful for posttraumatic symptoms. One possible reason is that the brain chemicals affected by these medications are related to both depressive symptoms and anxiety and posttraumatic symptoms. Another possible explanation is that the medications affect the posttraumatic symptoms that also are symptoms of depression, such as disrupted sleep, loss of motivation, and difficulty concentrating. Whatever the reason might be, research suggests that SSRIs can help survivors of trauma. In general, research on depression has shown that antidepressants are most helpful for those with severe depression, with effects for mild to moderate depression being negligible compared to placebo (inactive pills) (Fournier et al., 2009). Whether this is the case for PTSD is not known.

Prazosin

Recently, studies have begun to show benefits of a medication called **prazosin** (most common brand name Minipress), which has been used to treat high blood pressure for many years. Studies of veterans have shown that it can help reduce nightmares and sleep disturbances associated with PTSD. Prazosin can be extremely helpful for persons suffer-ing from nightmares and hyperarousal, because it directly turns down the systems in the body that are responsible for arousal. As such, it has a very different mechanism of action than antidepressants. Also, the effective dose can be quite variable, so whereas some may experience rapid relief, others may take many weeks to reach an effective dose. Unlike CBT, which can result in resolution of PTSD symptoms for the long term, the benefits of prazosin are present only while the medica-tion is being taken. In addition, some people experience lightheaded-ness and fainting upon standing up while they are taking prazosin. Although often this will resolve or can be managed by increasing the dose slowly, prazosin may not be suitable for everyone. Even so, pra-zosin appears to be one of the most effective tools we have for relatively rapid reduction in nightmares and improvement in sleep, although its utility for this purpose is not yet widely known among clinicians.

Novel Antipsychotics

There has been some research supporting the use of a group of medica-tions called **novel antipsychotics**, such as quetiapine (typically mar-keted as Seroquel) and risperidone (Risperdal), with trauma survivors diagnosed with PTSD. If your loved one is prescribed one of these med-ications, you may wonder why he's being given medication meant for patients with schizophrenia or bipolar disorder. These medications are sometimes used to enhance the effects of antidepressants. They also can improve reexperiencing symptoms, numbing/detachment, irrita-bility/anger, and sleep problems for some individuals with PTSD. These medications also can have effects on overall arousal similar to those of prazosin. These drugs have significant risks and side effects, however, so they may not be right for everyone.

Medications for Sleep Disturbances

Various medications can be prescribed to treat the sleep disturbances associated with PTSD. **Sedating antidepressants**, such as trazodone, are commonly used to facilitate sleep. Also, medications that treat insom-nia in the general population, such as zolpidem (marketed as Ambien), eszopiclone (Lunesta), and zaleplon (Sonata), are sometimes prescribed for PTSD-related sleep disturbances, although there is no research supporting their effectiveness when insomnia is associated with PTSD. **Benzodiazepines** are a class of medications that are sedating and that also reduce anxiety. There are numerous benzodiazepines, but the most commonly recognized ones are alprazolam (most common brand name Xanax), clonazepam (Klonopin), lorazepam (Ativan), and diazepam (Valium). Due to the high risk of serious side effects (e.g., cognitive impairment and worsening depression) and their potential for addiction, these medications are best reserved for short-term use (less than 1 month). Benzodiazepines were widely used to treat PTSD in the past, but their use has declined because research has failed to show effectiveness with PTSD and also because of the potential for addiction. Benzodiazepines are still used by some providers to treat the sleep problems associated with PTSD, but even as a sleep aid there is little evidence of benefits that would outweigh the risks. As discussed below, CBT for insomnia offers far more satisfactory resolution of insomnia in general, and this may be the case for PTSD-related insomnia as well. Sleep problems are so common among trauma survivors that we've included a separate section on treatment options below.

Treatments for Related Problems

As we discussed in Chapter 2, survivors of trauma often face a variety of difficulties in addition to PTSD. For example, besides numerous post-traumatic symptoms, Aaron had been quite depressed since returning from Afghanistan. Aaron's therapist considered that treatment of PTSD might improve Aaron's depression as well. But the fact that Aaron had had episodes of depression even before he went to Afghanistan pointed to the need for specific treatments for depression. Tess suffered from PTSD ever since the rape at school. But she also had struggled with an eating disorder since her early teens, which became much worse after the rape. So her parents, Maggie and Ian, weren't surprised that her bulimia continued even after her PTSD improved (more on eating disorders can be found later in this chapter). Tess's therapist planned a family meeting to discuss treatment options for this problem. Pamela had suffered from both PTSD and obsessive–compulsive disorder ever since she was molested by her babysitter when she was 10 years old. She was morbidly afraid of contamination and washed her hands so frequently that they were raw. Her fiancé, Caleb, couldn't understand why she never felt clean enough and was irritated that she expected him to wash so much too. Caleb wondered if her therapist had a plan to address the other effects the sexual abuse had had on her behavior. Most trauma survivors with PTSD have at least one additional problem, and these may or may not improve when PTSD improves. These problems may require treatment of their own, regardless of whether they are related to the trauma.

Depression

Depression affects as many as 60% of individuals with PTSD, and research suggests that it often improves when PTSD is treated. In cases where it doesn't, your loved one might benefit from behavioral activation, cognitive therapy, or interpersonal psychotherapy, all of which have been shown to be effective for depression. Little research has investigated the specific use of these treatments for depression that occurs with PTSD, but we've used these treatments clinically with good results. They also can help patients whose depression is so severe that it interferes with PTSD treatment. Behavioral activation presumes that depression is caused or exacerbated by withdrawal from life activities. Therapy focuses on helping the individual reengage with enjoyable life activities, particularly those that involve contact with others. Cognitive therapy entails learning to challenge negative thoughts that may contribute to depression. Interpersonal psychotherapy focuses on the role of relationships with others and their effect on mood. All of these are viable approaches for a person with PTSD and may benefit both PTSD and depression.

Anxiety Disorders

Anxiety disorders frequently co-occur with PTSD, including social anxiety, panic attacks, obsessions and compulsions, general worrying, health anxiety, and phobias. In fact, most patients with PTSD will have at least one additional anxiety disorder. Research has consistently shown that CBT is the treatment of choice for all such anxiety problems. In recent years the mounting evidence for the effectiveness of CBT for PTSD has led many therapists to seek training to provide this treatment, but that doesn't mean they have received training in conducting CBT for other problems, particularly related anxiety conditions. So if your loved one is troubled by additional anxiety problems, it may help to ask whether the therapist can provide CBT specifically for these other problems.

Sleep Problems

Sleep problems are among the most common complaints after trauma, which is why we've shown their many manifestations throughout this book so far. Your loved one may sleep better as his PTSD improves, as was the case for Marcus. While in Iraq, Marcus had slept barely a few hours every night due to the heat and noise of the generators and the possibility of nighttime ambushes. Back at home, he still felt on guard at night and hardly slept there either. He sometimes put his loaded gun under the bed to feel safer, but didn't tell Jenny because he knew it would upset her. After he started PTSD treatment he was better able to relax and his sleep improved.

Sleep doesn't always improve, however, after other posttraumatic stress symptoms resolve. Ever since Clare saw the uncle who had molested her at the family reunion, she had become more and more distant from her husband, Raj, and was so restless at night that some mornings Raj felt like she had beaten him up. It was at Raj's urging that she finally sought treatment for PTSD, and after several months many of her nightmares and other symptoms had improved. She wasn't as restless at night, but she still had a lot of trouble getting to sleep and looked exhausted all the time. She felt fatigued and irritable, and had lost interest in many of the activities she used to enjoy. Fortunately, there is a form of CBT specifically for insomnia, called CBT-I, that consists of several strategies that, if adhered to carefully, can improve sleep in 4 to 8 weeks. CBT-I includes methods for resetting the sleep cycle, learning to feel sleepy when in bed, and challenging thoughts and fears about *not* sleeping. Research consistently shows that for improving sleep for the long term, CBT-I is superior to medication, and it most certainly has fewer side effects. When Raj heard about CBT-I, he suggested that Clare ask her therapist about it. Her therapist referred her to another therapist who was trained in CBT-I methods. Although making changes in her sleep patterns was challenging at first, Clare started to fall asleep more quickly after a few weeks and within a few months slept through most nights. The effects on her daytime functioning were quite noticeable to both Clare and Raj: she snapped at him less, she had more energy to do fun things with him, and she was generally more cheerful. She was getting more done at work, too, which made her feel more effective.

Anger

Like disturbed sleep, problematic anger might resolve with treatment of PTSD. The interesting thing about anger is that it is part of the fight–flight response—anger is the flip side of fear, and in fact they are physiologically quite similar. This means that when a danger signal cues the survivor's fight–flight response, he can activate either emotion. Fear is equated with vulnerability and weakness, and therefore many people find fear an unpleasant or even unacceptable emotion to feel. Conversely, anger can be very empowering, and very often the trauma survivor is justified in feeling angry about the situation she endured.

A survivor who experiences both fear and anger in connection with the traumatic event may find it preferable to stay focused on the anger to avoid the powerlessness and vulnerability that goes with feeling afraid. For example, Chloe and her best friend were crossing the street when a drunk driver ran a red light and hit them. Chloe suffered extensive life-threatening injuries, including amputation of her arm, and she suffered headaches for years afterward. Her best friend was killed in the accident. Chloe was angry with the driver, and she was even angrier at the driver's lawyer and insurance company, who made it seem as if she and her friend were at fault. In the end, her settlement was barely enough to cover her medical bills, never mind that she was unable to work. Chloe's anger was justified, but it was there all the time, and it consumed her. She came to therapy only because her sister was concerned about how the anger was "eating away at her." In therapy, she learned how the anger interfered with processing the trauma memory and prevented her from reducing her fear. As long as she focused on anger, she avoided the fear. Her therapist taught her how to recognize anger and put it aside to focus on processing her fear. In the later stages of therapy, they worked on accepting changes in her life that resulted from the accident, and grieving the loss of her friend. Chloe also worked on strategies for channeling her anger into constructive activities, such as volunteering to assist groups lobbying for stricter drunk-driving laws.

In some cases, trauma-focused CBT may not be sufficient to resolve anger, especially anger that intrudes in daily life and leads to aggression or substance abuse. Although there is still much work to be done in developing effective methods of treating such anger problems, there are cognitive-behavioral approaches for anger management that are distinct from usual PTSD treatment. These methods offer important tools for some trauma survivors. In some cases it may be helpful to seek out a therapist who has this expertise.

Emotion Dysregulation

Another set of interventions that may be helpful for trauma survivors is treatment for emotion dysregulation. As discussed in Chapter 2, some trauma survivors lack skills for managing emotions and being effective in their relationships with others. These problems may warrant specific attention if they interfere with treatment of PTSD, are causing significant distress on their own, or pose a threat of harm to the survivor or others. A skilled therapist will be able to assess the problems carefully and advise whether to include specific treatment to help the survivor improve her skills for handling her emotional reactions and interacting in personal relationships. Fortunately, effective treatments are available for emotion dysregulation. Several forms of CBT, including a treatment called **dialectical behavior therapy**, can help persons who are struggling with long-standing social–emotional problems.

Alcohol and Other Substance Abuse

As noted in Chapter 2, many survivors of trauma use drugs or alcohol to avoid the painful memories and emotions associated with the trauma. For some survivors, the substance use is not severe and can be addressed in the course of treatment for PTSD. For example, Estelle told her therapist how much she had been drinking to get the memories out of her head. The therapist, taking into account her motivation for treatment and her lack of any history of substance abuse before the trauma, asked Estelle to refrain from drinking for the course of the therapy. They also agreed to monitor her drinking while she engaged in a trauma-focused treatment so that they could address any changes in reaction to the therapy activities. This system was helpful to Estelle.

Severe substance use, however, can cause significant problems in daily functioning or prevent adequate processing of the trauma memories, both of which can interfere with progress in therapy. If the substance use problem is severe, the therapist may suggest separate treatment for it before beginning trauma-focused therapy. When Jake started therapy, he was using cocaine a few times a week to deal with memories of being sexually abused as a child. Jake's therapist, who planned to provide exposure therapy, was concerned that Jake would use cocaine after sessions and after the homework activities, which would interfere with processing his feelings about the abuse and learning new information. So Jake and his therapist agreed that he would complete a course of substance abuse treatment and that they wouldn't start the exposure component of therapy until Jake was free of cocaine for 30 days.

A wide range of substance abuse treatments is available, and research has supported cognitive-behavioral substance abuse treatments, 12-step approaches (e.g., Alcoholics Anonymous or Narcotics Anonymous), and approaches that aim to increase the user's motivation to stop using ("motivational enhancement" therapy) as effective therapies. The relatively high frequency of substance use among survivors of trauma has led to development of approaches that treat substance use and PTSD at the same time. Research on one such dual treatment approach, called Seeking Safety (Najavits, 2002), has shown that it can help those with PTSD decrease their substance use and keep themselves safe.

Eating Disorders

Eating disorders can include episodes of binge eating, restriction of food intake, and various forms of purging, such as vomiting or excessive exercise. Preoccupation with food and body weight and shape also are hallmarks of eating disorders. Individuals who have a history of childhood sexual abuse are at greater risk for both eating disorders and PTSD. About 1 in 10 civilians seeking treatment for PTSD may have an eating disorder. Though less common than other problems, eating disorders complicate treatment significantly when they occur along with PTSD, as the two problems may be interrelated. Also, eating disorders are one of the most lethal psychiatric disorders, particularly among young women, who can suffer heart attacks or suicide due to the severe difficulties associated with eating disorders. A specific form of cognitive-behavioral therapy can help to reduce the binge–purge behavior associated with bulimia. When the eating disorder involves severe food restriction and weight loss, treatment is especially important, yet outcomes are less favorable. Few therapists have training in effective treatments for both eating disorders and PTSD. If your loved one is suffering from an eating disorder, referral to an eating disorder specialist may be necessary. In severe cases it may be necessary to address the eating disorder prior to treatment for PTSD, to prevent increasing frequency of dangerous behaviors during PTSD treatment.

You should now have a good idea of what types of therapy are available to help your loved one, but as we've made clear, it's not always easy to find a practitioner who is trained in effective therapies. What sorts of questions should you and your loved one ask as you choose a doctor or therapist? The next chapter guides you through this important process.

FIVE

Finding a Therapist

When Jim told Connie that he decided to go to therapy, she initially was excited, but then she started to have doubts. Sure, he had a lot of posttraumatic symptoms after being burned at work, but there was a lot of other stuff going on. He was drinking more than he used to, and there were also the physical injuries caused by the fire. He was in a lot of pain, and sometimes it seemed like that made him think more about the fire, and then he felt even more pain. Could one therapist help with all that? Connie wasn't so sure.

Doug tried to get his roommate, Will, to tell his doctor what was going on. Ever since Will saw that man get shot outside the club, he hadn't been the same. He wasn't sleeping right at all, and Doug was pretty sure he'd heard Will cry out during the night. He knew for sure that Will was drinking a lot more, and not in a social way. When he tried to broach the subject, Will told him he wasn't having any problems and he wasn't crazy. And, he said, there was no way he was going to tell a doctor that anything was going on, because it would get into his permanent record and he wanted to be a cop someday.

Juan was thrilled when Estelle came home and told him that she had let her gynecologist know what had happened to her and how much it was bothering her. Estelle said she was really relieved, because her gynecologist was understanding and supportive. She

even recommended a psychologist in the community who special-
ized in helping women who had been assaulted. But the psycholo-
gist was a man, and this made Estelle uncomfortable. How could
a man understand what she had gone through? And if the thera-
pist couldn't understand what she had been through, how could he
help? Juan didn't know what to say—she had never confided much
in him about the assault, and he wasn't sure he could understand
what she was concerned about.

Choosing a therapist is an important decision that can shape the course of your loved one's life. A trauma survivor who is stuck in his trauma and not moving forward with his life is like a person who doesn't know how to swim. He will have to tread water to prevent himself from drowning, but the more he treads, the more he feels like he's sinking. Though it will keep him alive, treading won't help him get to shore or to a boat. Even if he has someone like you in the water next to him to provide empathy and support to keep him from giving up, there won't be anyone to teach him to swim. The right therapist not only will be a supportive cheerleader but also a knowledgeable swim instructor. Finding such a person can make all the difference to your loved one for the rest of his life.

Finding the Right Therapist
and the Right Therapy

Many trauma survivors, especially those who have difficulty with trust, are focused on who the therapist is, whether they are comfortable with him and can trust him, and whether he seems to "get it." They may think that a therapist who has not gone through the specific traumatic experiences they have endured could not possibly understand them. This may be especially true for survivors who focus on their anger and feel as though the whole world is against them. These survivors may have difficulty believing that a well-intentioned mental health professional really does have their best interests in mind. Establishing comfort and trust is therefore essential to starting a therapy relationship that can lead to change. Talking about trauma, after all, entails disclosing some of the most intimate details of one's life experience. Moreover, deciding to talk about the trauma, rather than continuing to "stuff it away," requires that the trauma survivor trust the therapist's recommendation to do so.

There is a danger, however, that focusing on *who* is providing the therapy can result in paying insufficient attention to *what kind* of therapy the therapist will provide. As we discussed in Chapter 4, there is substantial evidence that structured trauma-focused therapies (those that involve the therapist guiding the client through trauma processing and fear reduction) are more effective than those that are primarily supportive or unstructured, or promote avoidance. By understanding the different kinds of therapy that are available, you will be better able to help your loved one find the right therapist, either by discussing this with him or by joining with him in interviewing potential therapists.

Given how scared Nadim had been, Wanda gave him some time to settle down, but she was intent on trying to help him make a decision about the kind of therapy he would pursue. She sometimes wondered whether something would be better than nothing, but she also remembered what she had read about how some treatments are more effective than others. So one evening, a week or so after the therapy session that really bothered him, Wanda brought up the topic of therapy again. Nadim wasn't as upset as he had been when he first got back from his therapy session, but he was still a little anxious about the prospect of talking about treatment again. He said that there was no way he was going back to that therapist; he didn't trust her. Wanda reminded him that she had been listed as an expert on a website, but Nadim was emphatic. So Wanda, seeking a compromise, suggested that instead of going back to the same therapist or avoiding treatment altogether, Nadim try another therapist on the list. Nadim thought about this and then said, "Well, I can try, but what if the next therapist tries to make me 'reexperience' the assault again?"

Wanda saw this as an opportunity to shift the focus from the therapist to the type of treatment. So she turned the question back to Nadim: "What if the second therapist suggests the same treatment? What would that tell us?" Nadim thought for a second, then his shoulders sagged in despair. "Well, if two of them say it, maybe that would mean it really could help. But how? I just don't get it!" Wanda confessed that she didn't either. So she didn't ask Nadim to agree to do anything before even seeing another therapist, but she did suggest that if the "reexperiencing" treatment came up again, he should ask the therapist why she would recommend that therapy and what its advantages and disadvantages were. Nadim sighed and agreed that this would be a reasonable plan. Wanda hoped that if Nadim focused on determining whether the therapy would work he would be less likely to find problems with the therapist.

The notion of interviewing potential therapists may come as a surprise to you. Many people do not consider that there are vast differences among therapists in their training, experience, expertise, approach, and comfort level with certain problems. It can be challenging to find a therapist who has the appropriate training and expertise in PTSD, is experienced and comfortable treating PTSD, and can manage the specific complicating issues involved. It's entirely possible that one person may not have all the necessary ingredients to treat all of your loved one's problems. When Clare first sought therapy, her husband, Raj, was concerned not only about PTSD and sleep problems but also about her eating. Ever since she saw her uncle at the family reunion, she had begun binge eating late at night, and she had gained 30 pounds. He guessed that this was somehow connected to the abuse she had suffered, but he had no idea how or what could help her. When they met with her therapist, they asked what could be done to help her with binge eating. The therapist explained that he was trained in cognitive-behavioral therapy for eating disorders. He suggested that, because the binge eating had begun simultaneously with the onset of PTSD, it might resolve after the PTSD was treated. If it did not, he would initiate CBT for binge eating. He explained that he preferred this sequential approach rather than trying to treat both problems at once, since doing so often feels overwhelming to the trauma survivor. As it turned out, the binge eating decreased dramatically after the PTSD treatment, although Clare's sleep did not improve. Her therapist did not have training in CBT-I (described in Chapter 4), so he referred her to another therapist for help with insomnia.

Most therapists are not trained in effective treatments for every possible problem trauma survivors might have. Think about all of the possible difficulties we listed in Chapter 2, and you can understand why. However, it's reasonable to expect a therapist to be familiar with the effective treatments for various problems and to formulate a plan for how the multiple problems your loved one is experiencing will be addressed. You can expect a good therapist to be candid about the limits of his training and expertise and to offer referrals to other professionals for problems that he does not have expertise in treating.

Getting Referrals

A good place to start in finding a CBT practitioner is for you or your loved one to ask your primary care provider. Talking with members of local support groups or asking mental health professionals that you already know for a referral also can help you identify potential therapists. Finally, useful resources for locating a therapist who is familiar with effective treatments for PTSD are national associations of cognitive-behavioral therapists and of trauma therapists, such as the Association of Behavioral and Cognitive Therapies (*www.abct.org*) or the International Society for Traumatic Stress Studies (*www.istss.org*). These organizations have databases of therapists that can help you locate therapists in your area. Being a member of one of these organizations does not guarantee the skill level of the therapist, but it does provide a higher level of assurance than simple licensure in a mental health profession. The Resources section at the back of this book contains contact information for these organizations and others in the United States and around the globe that can help you locate qualified therapists.

Interviewing Therapists

Efforts to locate a therapist might begin with a brief telephone conversation during which your loved one or you would seek to learn the basics of the therapist's training and expertise. Further discussion might occur in an initial meeting. Here are some things to ask.

What is your professional training/degree?

There are numerous avenues for training in psychotherapy or mental or behavioral health counseling, and it can help to know something about the background of different practitioners and what they do. At the least, the professional should have some form of training and license or certification in a bona fide mental health field. This provides assurance that the person meets minimum standards for providing therapy. It is not sufficient, however, to ensure that she is trained to provide evidence-based treatment for PTSD. In the United States, most providers of cognitive-behavioral therapy are clinical or counseling psychologists who have either a PhD (doctor of philosophy) or PsyD (doctor of psychology) degree because licensing laws in most U.S. states require a doctoral degree to practice as a psychologist. Many states have provisions for therapists to practice therapy with a master's degree as a social worker or "mental health" or "marriage and family" counselor. In a few states a psychologist can be licensed with a master's degree. In recent years, significant efforts have been under way to train master's-level therapists to practice CBT, especially for traumatized populations. This can include therapists who have an MSW (master's in social work) or a master's degree in counseling, marriage and family therapy, or other mental health field. For the most part, these degrees entail less rigorous training in skills for diagnosing mental health problems and delivering cognitive-behavioral therapy. This situation is improving, however, and many such therapists practice CBT quite competently based on training and experience they receive after they complete their degree. Note that in many other countries the master's degree or equivalent diploma is the primary degree for mental health practice. In these countries the doctoral degree is generally reserved for those who conduct research and/or teach at a university. Also, in some countries (e.g., Great Britain), psychiatric nurses and other counselor/therapists, who may have a bachelor's degree in nursing or counseling, receive extensive training in CBT and are common providers of effective psychotherapy.

Psychologists, social workers, and master's- and bachelor's-level counselors all specialize in psychotherapy and usually cannot prescribe medication. Usually (though not always) medications for PTSD will be prescribed by psychiatrists, who are medical doctors with specialized training in mental health. At a minimum, psychiatrists receive extensive training in prescribing medicines for emotional and behavioral disorders, and they receive general training in various forms of psychotherapy. Some psychiatrists receive additional training to specialize in CBT. So, although it is less common to find a psychiatrist who is highly skilled in CBT, there are some out there. Psychiatrists are not the only prescribers of medications for PTSD and related problems. Primary care providers, including medical doctors, physician assistants, and nurse practitioners, and some medical specialists, such as neurologists, physiatrists, pain specialists, and gastrointestinal specialists, often prescribe medications for depression and anxiety problems.

Psychology/Social Work Interns

Depending on where your loved one seeks treatment, she may be assigned to a psychology or social work intern. All trainees in psychology or social work are required to complete intensive clinical experiences before they are awarded their degree. Many civilian or Veterans Affairs medical centers have internship programs where licensed psychologists and social workers provide regular supervision for interns completing their degrees. Interns usually have finished their classroom studies and are learning how to put what they know into practice. People have mixed feelings about receiving treatment from interns. Some trauma survivors want to be treated by experienced professionals and refuse to be assigned to interns. Other trauma survivors prefer interns because they believe that, having recently completed their schooling, they have more current knowledge than a supervisor who trained 25 years ago. If your loved one is referred to an intern, he can ask her the same questions we outline here. In addition, he should ask who her supervisor is. He can even ask to meet with her supervisor to assess the supervisor's experience in treating posttraumatic problems and supervising interns.

They may refer to a psychiatrist only when the patient's response to those treatments is not optimal. Very often, talking with a primary care clinician or other doctor may be the first place your loved one goes for help, and this person may be able to provide a referral for CBT.

What is your approach to therapy?

Your aim in asking this question is to find out what specific therapy modalities (e.g., CBT, interpersonal therapy, psychodynamic therapy, and supportive therapy) the clinician practices. Many therapists who treat trauma survivors identify themselves as "eclectic." This means that they utilize many different forms of therapy and select the methods they think will suit a particular client and her problems. They may practice a wide variety of methods for healing PTSD, some of which have not been demonstrated effective through research. If you really want your loved one to "get better," keep in mind that your chances of getting good results from therapy are greater if the therapist uses methods that have been proven effective through research. If a therapist describes his approach as eclectic, it can be useful to ask for more specifics about the types of interventions he uses, what he views as the major aims of therapy for PTSD (look for mention of processing the trauma or anxiety reduction), and how he decides which strategies to employ.

How familiar are you with effective treatments for PTSD?

The more familiar your loved one and you are with the treatments, the better you will be able to interpret how the therapist responds to this question. You might find some therapists who speak of the treatment they do as being effective in their own experience. It's important to realize that a clinician's experience with a treatment is not the same strength of evidence as research demonstrating a treatment's effect. Also, you should be skeptical of a therapist who promises or guarantees effective results. Even the treatments supported by research are not effective 100% of the time, particularly when there are complicating factors in your loved one's situation. A responsible therapist will speak candidly about the limits of his specific skills and knowledge as well as the limits of what therapy can do.

How much experience have you had using these treatments with PTSD?

From an ethical standpoint, a therapist should be honest about his level of experience. Although extensive experience with specific treatments for PTSD is not essential to be helpful, a therapist who has had more experience may be more familiar with areas of difficulty in treatment and might have more tools at her disposal for resolving therapy impasses. Conversely, she might be very experienced in treating trauma survivors, but new to using CBT. If this is the case, she might be receiving consultation from another colleague to guide her. This could be helpful in treating your loved one, and it is something you have a right to know about.

Can you also help with [insert your loved one's other problem]?

As discussed in Chapter 4, many of the problems that co-occur with PTSD have defined, effective treatments. If your loved one has specific other problems that you know of, it will be helpful to know whether those can be addressed by this therapist. For example, many patients with PTSD suffer from depression and other anxiety disorders. Does this therapist have experience conducting the treatments for these problems?

How do you come up with a treatment plan?

Regardless of the therapist's level of experience, you will want to know something about how she gathers information about your loved one's problems and comes up with a "formulation." A formulation is the therapist's theory about what is causing the problems and why they continue. A thorough formulation should look at all of the survivor's problems and how they are connected. A good formulation gives your loved one and the therapist the best chance of developing a treatment plan that will work. A skilled CBT therapist will share all her ideas and thoughts about the problems your loved one faces. She will work collaboratively with him to come up with a formulation that makes sense to both of them. The therapist will explain how the formulation leads to the treatment plan. She will seek feedback from the survivor and from you and other important people in the survivor's life to make sure everyone is in agreement before proceeding.

The formulation might prove to be completely correct, but a good therapist will have in mind alternative theories and ideas about how the plan might change if the formulation does not bear out in treatment. For example, Clare's therapist was aware of her sleep problem and considered the possibility that the PTSD symptoms were causing the sleep disruption. He knew research shows that about half of patients will sleep better after their PTSD is treated. If Clare's sleep did not improve, it would suggest that something else might be influencing her sleep, in which case the therapist was prepared to refer her for CBT-I. It's not essential that you know *all* the theories and alternative plans, but it's useful to have a sense of how the therapist comes up with them. Also, it's important that the therapist collaborate with your loved one to develop a treatment plan and make any modifications to it. It's always a good sign when the therapist begins treatment with a thorough assessment of your loved one's experiences and the various problems that interfere with daily life.

How are family and other loved ones involved in therapy?

A good therapist will allow and encourage family members or loved ones to participate in treatment, especially during the initial phases. The more you understand about what is happening in therapy and why, the more you can support the process and help your loved one make positive changes. You can contribute by reminding your loved one about the homework assignments, talking with her about obstacles to doing them, or even doing some of them, such as *in vivo* exposure, with her. If she is doing imaginal exposure, it's usually best to encourage your loved one to do the homework but not listen to the recordings yourself—the material may be highly personal or graphic and upsetting. Your loved one might feel uncomfortable or ashamed disclosing details of the trauma to you, especially in the early phase of therapy. Also, usually it isn't helpful if you become distraught about specific aspects of the memory. The therapist will indicate if there is a time when it can be therapeutic for your loved one to share the specifics of the trauma with you. Otherwise, it may be best kept private. If you notice that your loved one avoids doing therapy assignments, you might consider talking with him about the effects of his avoidance (as in decision analysis; see Chapter 3) and pointing out how the assignments might benefit him in the long run. You can be an important cheerleader and even a coach for your loved one as he does this difficult work.

Questions for a Potential Therapist

- "What is your professional training/degree?"
- "What is your approach to therapy?"
- "How familiar are you with effective treatments for PTSD?"
- "How much experience have you had using these treatments with PTSD?"
- "Can you also help with [loved one's problem]?"
- "How do you come up with a treatment plan?"
- "How are family and other loved ones involved in therapy?"

Realistic Expectations

When Aaron finally agreed to see a therapist at the VA, Julie went in with him. The therapist seemed really nice, although she wasn't much older than Aaron and Julie. She talked about how treatment is about more than just coping with the trauma. She explained that treatment is about processing the memories and emotions and living a full, valued life. This sounded great to Julie, and her first question was, "Will he ever be the person he used to be?" The therapist smiled and said this was an understandable hope, but that no treatment could undo the effects of time and experience. Aaron would be forever changed in different ways by his experiences in Afghanistan, but these changes would not necessarily have to interfere with his life or negatively affect his relationship with Julie. Julie still wished she could have her old husband back, but she could understand. Aaron had had some amazing experiences. Of course he would be affected by them. Eventually, Aaron and Julie came to realize, as well, that not all of the effects were negative. (We talk more about how this happens in Chapter 12.)

Finding the right therapist to deliver the most effective therapy will not change your loved one back to how she was before the trauma, and it won't guarantee that her symptoms will disappear. But it will provide the best chance for her to be able to live her life without interference from the trauma and for you to strengthen your relationship and move forward in your lives together.

What If My Loved One Doesn't Improve at All with Treatment?

Unfortunately, there is always a chance that your loved one won't experience improvements from treatment. In that case, what can you do?

First, it's important to realize that therapy in general requires committing time and effort to change many parts of life for the better. Therapy for PTSD can be especially difficult. For most trauma survivors, facing memories of frightening or horrific events is hard work, and some people are reluctant to feel the uncomfortable emotions that it can bring up. Some people do not feel ready to tackle this task. The potential gains do not seem to outweigh the discomfort they may feel in the process, not to mention the time, inconvenience, effort, and possibly the financial costs of attending regular therapy sessions. Some people, especially those who have put a lot of effort into avoiding thinking about the trauma, find that memories, dreams, and distress

increase during the early phase of therapy. This is a sign that processing has begun and does not mean that the therapy will not work. Yet
in some cases the increased reexperiencing of trauma memories leads
the person to stop therapy.

If your loved one has started therapy and dropped out, you might
gently initiate a discussion of the costs and potential benefits of resuming therapy. This would be an excellent time to use the decision analysis
tool we talked about in Chapter 3. You can start a new form to examine
the potential pros and cons of resuming therapy. Or, if you had already
listed them for the initial decision to start therapy, you could use that
as a starting point and add any new factors that have come up. If there
are newly discovered obstacles, such as transportation, child care, or
scheduling limitations, you might help the survivor generate ways to
overcome them. As tempted as you may be to pressure the survivor
or demand that he stick with therapy, try not to do so. Usually, the
harder we push people to change, the harder they push back against
us. Instead, offer observations. When Nadim stopped going to his therapy sessions, Wanda found a time when they were alone together and
said, "I've noticed you've been withdrawn from me and the kids lately.
It seems like you're still really bothered by the mugging. I wonder if
dealing with it on your own is working out for you."

If your loved one did not show improvement after a reasonable
amount of therapy, there are several options to consider. It may be
appropriate for you and your loved one to meet with the therapist
together to discuss his progress. The important question is whether
more of the same kind of therapy is likely to help. Sarah was in
therapy for 6 months with a therapist who worked with her using
present-focused problem-solving therapy. During this time, her mood
improved, and she was managing her daily stress much better. However, she still feared and avoided public places and continued to have
nightmares about the assault. At this point the therapist recommended
transferring her treatment to a therapist who was an expert in CBT.

Paul had worked with his therapist at the VA using a form of CBT
called cognitive processing therapy. After several months of therapy he
was much less bothered by his guilt about shooting the child. However,
he continued to show strong startle reactions and sometimes felt suddenly panicked when he saw children, or any of several other reminders of his time in Iraq. He also continued to avoid many public places

Self-Help and Internet-Based Treatment

What if my loved one can't or won't go for therapy—can he help himself using an Internet program or self-help book?

It's no secret that for certain groups of trauma survivors, such as military service members and veterans, police, and fire and rescue workers, there is stigma associated with having PTSD. Many such trauma survivors are reluctant to seek help. They may be concerned that if they are struggling with intrusive memories, anxiety, irritability, and the like, others will see them as weak or damaged. They may fear that others, particularly "higher-ups" at work, will find out about the problems they are having and that this will affect their work status. Or they may simply be resistant to disclosing painful experiences with a therapist. Other trauma survivors might be willing to go for therapy, but they face practical or financial obstacles to obtaining effective therapy. They may have difficulty locating a skilled trauma therapist, be unable to fit therapy into their schedules, or have trouble with transportation to appointments. For those who are unable, unwilling, or simply not ready to seek therapy, brochures, books, and online materials can be a good starting point for trauma survivors seeking information about trauma and PTSD. As a substitute for therapy, however, they are less likely to be of value. Unfortunately, the two studies to date that have looked at whether reading a self-help book improved PTSD found that it did not, despite the fact that the self-help books discussed cognitive-behavioral strategies. It seems that reading and acquiring knowledge is not sufficient to help a person put changes in coping skills to work in day-to-day life. Internet-based interventions might be more promising as they can offer more guidance to the survivor in applying the strategies. Several studies have suggested that programs that guide the trauma survivor through writing about the traumatic experience can be helpful. Yet the availability of such programs remains limited. No English-language programs to guide writing or other forms of exposure are as yet widely available on the Internet. This area is developing at a rapid pace, however, and it is likely that in the future we will see more Internet-based treatments and, eventually, research informing us about their effectiveness.

out of fear of seeing children. His therapist, who was trained primarily in cognitive processing therapy, decided to refer him to another therapist who could provide prolonged exposure therapy.

Freddie had been in therapy for years after being pinned by the forklift at work. His therapists had been terrific. They were highly supportive and taught him meditation skills to help him relax and be less stressed and more focused in his daily life. However, he still was bothered by loud noises, feared leaving his house, had nightmares, and slept just a few hours each night. During an independent medical evaluation requested by the workers' compensation company, it was pointed out that Freddie had not had a trial of exposure therapy, so he was referred to a therapist who could provide this. If one treatment approach has not worked, it's worth getting another opinion and looking at treatments that have not been tried.

As we've mentioned, your loved one may have tried to engage in some form of trauma-focused CBT but found the treatment too difficult to tolerate. Experts in traumatic stress may be able to work at figuring out whether particular changes to the treatment, alternative interventions, or medication might make the treatment more tolerable. Janine started trauma-focused CBT beginning with cognitive therapy. With the focus on her trauma-related thoughts, her nightmares increased, and she found she couldn't function when she was sleeping only 3 hours per night. Her therapist suggested a trial of medication for nightmares. Within a few weeks, the nightmares became less disturbing and she was sleeping 7 hours per night. She subsequently was able to engage in exposure therapy to reduce her overall PTSD. Jim completed a full course of exposure therapy that focused on the memory of the fire at work. He experienced significant reduction of PTSD symptoms and his nightmares decreased in frequency, but they did not fully remit. In reviewing his progress, his therapist offered two options that might help to reduce his nightmares further: the medication prazosin or imagery rehearsal therapy (see Chapter 4). In cases where the survivor is unable or unwilling to attempt exposure therapy, imagery rehearsal therapy, which targets nightmares specifically and is less effective for overall PTSD, might be helpful from the start.

The key is not to give up on finding the right help. Review options with the therapist and pursue a second (or even a third) opinion when symptoms don't improve after a reasonable course of therapy, and certainly if there has been no progress within 6 months to a year. And never be afraid to consider a new therapist who has experience with therapeutic approaches your loved one has not yet tried.

Traumatic events can have profound effects on those who survive them. For those with chronic PTSD, change is unlikely without some form of intervention. The good news is that PTSD itself can often be resolved with 3 to 6 months of weekly therapy, as long as your loved one commits to being fully engaged in the therapy both during and outside of therapy sessions. The actual time frame in which your loved one is in therapy might be longer if she requires treatment for other problems in addition to PTSD, if she is not fully committed to therapy, or if life just gets in the way of therapy. Especially if the survivor in your life has taken a significant time to agree to start therapy, it can be disheartening to face the possibility that he'll drop in and out of therapy and stretch out this time frame. That's one of the many reasons it's so important that you not only try to help your loved one but also take care of yourself, the subject of the next chapter.

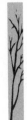

PART II

Helping Yourself, Helping the Survivor

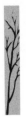

SIX

Taking Care of Yourself

Juan didn't want his wife to be alone. When Estelle lay awake at night, he stayed up with her, often telling her stories to try to keep her mind occupied so she could fall asleep. If she got nervous at the last minute before a party or event and decided she couldn't go, Juan would make up a story and cancel so he could stay home with her. In fact, because Estelle didn't like to leave the house and didn't feel safe alone, Juan stayed home with her almost all the time. He stopped playing with his softball team and went running less and less frequently. After a while, he noticed he had less energy and wasn't as interested in activities that he used to enjoy.

Bill couldn't stand the idea of turning his daughter out of the house, but he wasn't sure that he and Mattie could go on living with her. Wendy was up at all hours of the night and was irritable all day. Mattie had cut down to part-time at work to stay with her, but this didn't seem to help. Ever since the fire, Wendy had been getting steadily worse and more reclusive, and it seemed like she was taking him and Mattie with her. They had to start taking better care of themselves, or they would really be headed for trouble.

Zach's brother Hank drank way too much after he got out of the military, and after bailing him out of jail twice, Zach decided it was easier to go out with him and make sure he didn't get into too much trouble. After a couple of weeks, Zach was feeling really run down.

He wasn't getting a lot of sleep because of the late nights. And he would never have guessed that sneaking into work late without having showered would make him feel so gross. But it did.

Given all the ways that trauma can affect a person, it's understandable that you want to help the trauma survivor in your life. But your caring and concern can have the unintended side effect of draining you of the resources you need to care for yourself. If your efforts to support the trauma survivor in your life are hurtful to you, you may end up less helpful than you otherwise would have been. We want to minimize any suffering you might be going through and help you stay as healthy as possible during this difficult time. In this chapter, we take you through different ways to make sure you're taking good care of yourself as well as your loved one.

How Do You Know If You're Not Taking Care of Yourself?

When we discussed the various types of stressful events in Chapter 2, we noted that stress affects different people in different ways. The same can be said about the effects of caring for a trauma survivor. For example, Bill and Mattie had raised three children in a tough, poor area of the city, and they had always been able to smile about their struggles. When their daughter, Wendy, moved back in with them after she was badly injured in a fire in the factory where she worked, they were able to slip right back into their parenting mindset and care for Wendy without missing a day of work. After 8 months, when she was back on her feet physically and had gotten treatment for the nightmares and intense anxiety she had been feeling, they helped her find an apartment. When Wendy was finally settled into her own place and had started a new job, Bill and Mattie went back to their own routines. In contrast Wallace, whose wife, Maria, was having problems readjusting to the civilian world after her tour in Afghanistan, found himself worrying about her to the point where it interfered with his job. After seeing Wallace for the fourth time in 3 months, his primary care doctor finally recommended that he try counseling to get help.

How has your concern about the trauma survivor in your life affected you? You may be coping well with the additional strain, or it may be taking a toll on you. Pay attention to your mind and body and look for signs of stress and poor self-care. Take notice of how well you are fulfilling your obligations—falling behind at work or on bills, not keeping your living space clean, or failing to take care of basic needs such as showering or brushing your teeth may be signs that you are not taking adequate care of yourself. Signs that you have been struggling with stress for a long period of time include:

- Difficulty falling or staying asleep
- Low energy
- Loss of interest in activities you used to enjoy
- Loss of motivation to complete basic tasks
- Hard time concentrating or focusing attention
- Muscle aches and pains
- Changes in eating (eating more or eating less)
- Sad or irritable mood
- Racing thoughts/excessive worry
- Restlessness/agitation
- Increase in physical complaints/problems
- Thoughts about death or dying

If you notice yourself having any of these problems, they may signal that you should focus less on the trauma survivor and more on your own well-being. Follow the recommendations in this chapter to ensure that you're taking adequate care of yourself.

You may feel conflicted about prioritizing yourself above someone who has been traumatized and can't meet his own needs. But keep in mind that if you're not taking adequate care of yourself, you really won't be able to devote much energy to your loved one. It's like being instructed on a plane to put on your own oxygen mask before your child's: if you pass out while trying to put on your child's mask, neither of you will get the air you both need. If you want to help a trauma survivor, you have to make sure you're functioning at your best to provide the best support for your loved one.

You don't have to "gut it out," sacrificing your own needs and well-being to help the person you care about. You can meet some of your own needs while taking care of those of the trauma survivor. In Chapter 7, we talk about how to determine what you're willing to do for the trauma survivor and make sure you are taking care of yourself.

But for now, keep in mind that you have a right to take care of yourself, and it's best for both you and the survivor that you make sure your basic needs are met. If not, you may run yourself into the ground while your ability to support your loved one steadily declines.

The Basics

During times of increased stress, we often have trouble getting our most basic needs met. Things like diet, sleep, and even hygiene can fall by the wayside as we focus on what is stressing us. We tell ourselves that we'll eat later or catch up on sleep once the struggle is over. What most of us don't realize, unfortunately, is that times of great stress are when we most need to sleep and eat well. Our bodies depend on rest and energy. Not eating well literally deprives the body of energy it needs, and so it actually becomes harder to deal with problems. The same is true for sleep. There is a reason your grandmother used to tell you to "get a good night's sleep" before you had to do something important. When we're sleepy, we're more likely to be irritable, have difficulty concentrating, and make poor decisions.

Eating

Most of us know the fundamentals of healthy eating, so we'll just give you some quick reminders here. There are numerous sources of nutritional information and quick and healthy recipes and meal plans that you can seek out. Keep in mind that the two important aspects of eating are what you eat and when you eat. The healthier you eat, the more energy you will have and the clearer your head will feel. Edna noticed that she was eating a lot of fast food because she was spending so much time with her son Brett, making sure he got to his appointments at the VA. After a few weeks, she noticed that her energy level was low and she had gained weight. She couldn't believe that changing her diet could affect those things so quickly, but it did.

Research shows that when we eat on a regular schedule, our bodies will want to maintain that routine. In other words, if you're used to eating lunch at noon every day while at work, you will probably want to eat lunch around noon on the weekends too, even if there's nothing in your schedule that compels you to do so. In contrast, when we skip meals or eat on a very irregular schedule, our energy level can drop and our hunger and fullness cues can get disrupted. Also, poor eating is related to poorer health overall, as well as weight gain.

There is clear evidence that the type of food you eat can have a significant effect on overall health and well-being. If your diet consists of healthy, low-fat, high-fiber foods, you're more likely to feel better overall and have fewer health problems and more energy. If your diet consists of low-quality fatty foods, you will not feel as good. Unfortunately, the foods that are bad for you are usually the simplest ones to get. It's easier to grab something "on the run" from a drive-through to fill up than to set aside time to cook healthy food.

Ideally you should eat three meals, at the usual breakfast, lunch, and dinner times, plus two or three light snacks each day. Here are a few suggestions for fitting them into your life:

- Fill your grocery list with healthy food, not junk.
- Spend a few minutes each morning reviewing your day's schedule and plan accordingly. If Edna knew that Brett had an appointment at the VA and she would be there for several hours, she made sure to toss an apple or a banana into her bag so that she'd have a healthy snack; if the appointment was in the middle of the day, she would pack a sandwich for lunch.
- Make sure you always have the ingredients for a few quick meals on hand. When Edna got home late, she could throw together a healthy meal quickly with ingredients she kept in her cupboard and freezer.
- When you have time to cook, make extra and refrigerate or freeze it. On nights when there was no time to cook, Edna always had some leftover meatloaf and veggies from the fridge that she could heat up. And she discovered that no food tastes as good as the food you didn't cook that night!

As for *what* you eat:

- Focus on ways to eat vegetables, fruits, whole-grain foods, beans, nuts, and lean meats like fish or chicken.
- Try to stay away from fatty meats and sweets.
- Don't forget that what you drink is an important part of your diet. Make sure you drink enough water during the day and try to stay

away from less healthy beverages (like sodas) and limit your caffeine intake to a reasonable amount.

Sleep

We've already given many examples of how sleep—yours and the survivor's—can be disrupted by the symptoms of trauma when you sleep in the same bed or even the same house. But your sleep may be affected by the trauma survivor in your life even if he doesn't live in your house, simply because you're worried about him. Wayne assured his father, Bob, that he was fine. He always told Bob not to worry about him, even after a second DUI, a third job loss, and the end of his marriage, all within a year after he had returned from the Gulf War. But Bob knew that his son was still suffering from his combat experience. At night, when his mind was finally free of the day's business and he lay down to go to sleep, worries about his son would take over his thoughts. During times of stress it can be harder to fall asleep, and even when we do fall asleep we may be disturbed by troubling dreams.

There are three keys to sleeping well: keeping a regular schedule, not staying in bed when you're awake, and making sure your bedroom is an environment conducive to sleep. Here are some ideas for all three:

• Keep your wake time constant during the week and don't sleep more than an hour later on the weekend.

• Even if your sleep schedule is not within your control, you can control what you do once you get off schedule. Get back to your routine as soon as you can and also resist the temptation to make up for lost sleep, which will only keep you off schedule.

• If you're not sleepy, do not get into bed, even if it's your bedtime.

• If you lie awake in bed for more than 15 minutes, get out of bed and do something quiet, such as reading a book or magazine or doing crossword puzzles or sudoku, until you are sleepy. When your head starts to nod, return to bed.

• If worrying is keeping you awake at night, a few hours before bedtime devote 15 or 20 minutes to writing down all the things that are on your mind. Next to each thing you have been worrying about, write down what you can do about it next and plan when you will do it. If it is something you can take care of right then and there, do it. If you have been trying to remember to pay a bill, and you have the money, then pay the bill so it's off your mind. If there is nothing you can do about the problem at that moment, then plan your next step and write it down. This way your mind has an easier time putting that worry aside at bedtime. When you schedule time to "worry" about your problems in a systematic way prior to bedtime, it's less likely that those concerns will be running through your head when it's time to sleep.

• Adjust the light, noise level, and temperature to suit your preferences (most people find they sleep better in a dark, quiet, and cool room).

• If you and the trauma survivor have different sleep preferences, the two of you will have to work out how the sleep environment will be set up. We talk more about how to be assertive to get your needs met in Chapter 8. If, however, there is no way to adjust the light, noise, or temperature to suit you both, then sleeping separately may be the best short-term solution.

Exercise

Exercise can increase your energy level, improve your sleep, enhance concentration and memory, and protect you from illnesses—all of great benefit when you're feeling the stress of trying to help a trauma survivor. Unfortunately, when you're anxious about different issues in your life, it can be even more difficult than usual to wrangle the time and motivation necessary to exercise. Here are some ideas for getting beneficial exercise even though you're devoting a lot of time and energy to the trauma survivor in your life:

• Consider something as simple as devoting 25 minutes per day to taking a brisk walk (for the average person that would mean covering about a mile to a mile and a half). This would total more than 150 minutes of moderate activity in a week, the amount recommended by the Centers for Disease Control and Prevention (otherwise known as the CDC) for moderate physical activity for adults.

• Also engage in muscle-strengthening activities at least twice a week for about 20 minutes—working out with weights, working against your body's own resistance (e.g., push-ups or pull-ups), doing yoga, or participating in strenuous outdoor work like digging holes or shoveling snow.

- If you work on a high floor, taking the stairs up to your office in the morning and after lunch will provide you with about 10 minutes of moderate exercise a day.
- Parking as soon as you get into the lot and then walking the rest of the way to the store (and back) can provide another 5 to 10 minutes of walking (and can save you the headache of searching for a spot).

Often loved ones feel guilty if they leave the trauma survivor alone. Greg felt this way about his girlfriend, Jeanette, after she was mugged. But he started feeling sluggish and irritable after giving up his regular basketball games, so he compromised by deciding to play basketball again on Saturdays, promising to keep his cell phone in his pocket, and confined the rest his exercise to lifting weights, doing calisthenics, and jumping rope in the garage.

Relaxation

As we noted in Chapter 1, you may be feeling anxious, sad, angry, and helpless as you try to live with and help the trauma survivor in your life. After an argument that seemed to come out of nowhere you walk around with your fists clenched and your stomach in knots. Or you may notice that after your loved one nearly jumps out of his seat for the fourth time in the movie theater your heart is racing and you're sweating too. You may worry about her a lot, which makes you anxious and sad. The stress of all these emotions can make it hard for you to focus on what you have to do and how you want to live. For some, living with a trauma survivor can lead to stress-related health problems, such as headaches, stomachaches or irregular bowels, muscle aches, poor sleep, and fatigue.

Our bodies and minds cannot sustain the accelerated pace you might be keeping to take care of the survivor in your life—we eventually need to stop and take a break or we will exhaust ourselves. Relaxation is a valuable skill that can help you pause amid the rush of all the things you're trying to do and ease your stress. Regular relaxation practice offers you a break from daily tensions and an opportunity to recover. Taking as little as 10 minutes each day at a specific time to relax and refresh yourself can help you be better prepared for what's ahead of you. Relaxation also can be applied in stressful situations when you're feeling anxious or upset as a way to calm yourself so that you're better able to do what you have to do.

You may find it surprisingly difficult to let up on yourself and take a break. Relaxation takes practice, so if it seems like it's not working at first, don't give up. Much like with sleep and exercise, you may find yourself thinking, "I have no time for this! This will prevent me from doing other things!" And much like sleep and exercise, relaxation is an activity whose rewards make the time investment well worth it.

There are many ways to relax. We'll explain the most common ones, and we recommend that you try out each one to find out what works best for you. For most of us, these are new skills, so it may take time to learn them. Don't give up! The more you practice, the better you'll get.

Breathing-Based Relaxation

Focusing on your breathing to facilitate relaxation is a very old tradition. One of the advantages of breathing-based relaxation is that wherever we go our breath is with us, so we can use this type of relaxation in just about any situation. Breathing-based relaxation focuses on changing the rate of breathing as well as the way we breathe. When you slow down your breathing and breathe in a deeper, more rhythmic way, your whole body tends to slow down along with it, and you will feel more relaxed.

When your body is aroused, you take fast, short, sharp breaths and exhale quickly. Your chest moves visibly in this type of breathing. In contrast, when relaxing, try to breathe using your *diaphragm*. The diaphragm is a membrane of muscle that sits below your lungs. When the diaphragm contracts, it increases the volume of your lungs and draws air into them, much like the way a fireplace bellows sucks in air when you open it. When you breathe using your diaphragm, your stomach moves more than your chest and your breaths are slower and deeper. Some people refer to this as "baby breathing." If you have ever watched a small baby sleeping, its belly moves as it breathes, much like a little balloon inflating and deflating. This is the same slow, rhythmic breathing that can help you to relax. When breathing slows, you take in less air and the amount of oxygen in your blood decreases, slowing your heart rate and leading to an overall relaxation of the body.

The steps for diaphragmatic breathing are simple:

1. Sit in a comfortable chair with your feet on the floor and your arms at rest. If you like, place one hand on your chest and the other on your belly. If you're comfortable closing your eyes, close them. If not, stare at a blank spot on the wall or the floor.
2. Breathe in normally through your nose. There's no need to take a very deep breath.
3. Exhale slowly through your mouth. Take several breaths this way.
4. As you continue to breathe, start to slow your breathing down. After you exhale, count silently to three before your next inhalation.
5. As you continue to breathe, try to pay attention to each breath. Notice how the air is cool and dry as it enters your nose and then moist and warm as it flows out through your mouth.
6. If you notice your attention going to something other than your breath, that's okay. Just bring the focus back to the air and continue to breathe.

Try breathing like this twice a day for about 10 minutes each time. Don't be discouraged if it's difficult at first, or even if breathing this way seems to make you more nervous than you were before you started. Just keep practicing focusing your attention on your breath. You'll find that the more you breathe this way at home, sitting down, with your eyes closed, the better you will be at breathing this way standing up in line at the grocery store or driving in traffic with your eyes wide open.

Muscle-Based Relaxation

Some people find it more effective to relax by decreasing the tension in their body. When we're under stress, our muscles tighten up and remain tense, which can result in muscle aches. We may not notice this as it's happening. For example, your shoulders and neck may be tense all day, but you may not realize it until later at night when you try to settle down to rest and find that your shoulders are sore.

Muscle-based relaxation involves tensing and relaxing the major sets of muscles in your body. As you tense, hold, and then release and relax each muscle group, you pay attention to what the tension feels like, so that you may be more likely to notice tension in that body part later on. Over time, you may start to notice that certain parts of your body tend to be tense more than others. If so, you can focus your attention on relaxing these particular areas.

The box below describes the different muscle groups in your body and how to tense and relax them. For each muscle group, follow these steps:

1. Tense the muscle group hard, but without causing pain.
2. Hold for a count of five, paying attention to the tension and what it feels like.
3. Slowly let the tension out of the muscles, letting them rest easy.
4. Pay attention to the lack of tension in the muscles, and what it feels like.

Muscle Relaxation

Muscle group	How to tense that muscle group
Lower legs	With knees straight and feet sticking out in front of you, tense your ankles and lower legs so that your toes curl up toward your nose.
Upper legs	Try to raise yourself off your chair by tensing your buttocks and the backs of your thighs.
Stomach	Suck in your tummy as far as you can.
Lower arms	With your palms down, make a fist and then pull the back of your fist back toward your forearm.
Upper arms	Without tensing your lower arms, pull your elbows and inner upper arms in toward your sides.
Chest	With your shoulders back, take a deep breath and stretch your chest out.

Shoulders	Shrug your shoulders up toward your ears.
Neck	Tilt your head back slightly and thrust your chin out in front of you so that you feel the tension in the back of your neck.
Lower face	Purse your lips and pull back the corners of your mouth.
Upper face	Frown.
Head	Raise your eyebrows as far as you can, feeling the tension in the top of your head.

As with breathing, the more you practice this exercise at home when you're comfortable, the more easily you'll be able to tense and relax your muscles when you are feeling stressed. As you get better and better at muscle-based relaxation, you'll find that instead of having to tense and relax your lower legs and then your upper legs, you can do both at once. Next you may practice simply recalling the tension and allowing relaxation to occur. With practice, you'll start to notice the tension in your muscles more often, so that you can employ muscle relaxation when you need it most. In addition to the physical benefits of releasing muscle tension, muscle relaxation teaches you to shift your mental focus away from worrisome thoughts and images. Many people find that, if practiced shortly before bedtime, it helps sleep. Focusing on your muscles can draw your attention away from worrying about how your loved one is doing, fretting about how much work you have to do, rehashing a recent argument, or other mental activity that interferes with sleep.

Imagery- or Sound-Based Relaxation

Instead of focusing your attention on your breath as in the diaphragmatic breathing exercise, you might try focusing on a picture or a mental image of a safe, comfortable, calming place. Focusing on the image and its pleasant characteristics can help you relax. The image might be of a place you've been to and really liked, such as a beautiful beach on a tropical island, or a place you loved as a child, such as a clubhouse or a park, or just an inviting scene such as the forest picture from the calendar on your wall. Whatever you choose, it should be a scene that does not have anything negative associated with it.

To use imagery to relax, find a quiet place and make yourself comfortable. Close your eyes and take a few slow breaths to steady yourself. Then picture your safe place in as much detail as you can. Try to picture every aspect of the scene. For example, if you are on a warm, sunny beach, try to focus on the color of the sand, the fronds of the palm trees, the hairs on the coconuts, and the color of the water. Focus, as well, on sounds, smells, and sensations, such as the sound of the waves crashing, the smell of salt air, and the feeling of sun warming your skin. Then, if your safe place is big enough, take yourself on a tour of it. Walk along the beach, feeling the cool, wet sand and occasionally the water washing over your feet.

Focusing your attention on a particular type of sound that you find soothing or relaxing also can draw your attention away from what is making you anxious. Some people find natural sounds very pleasant. Recordings of forest or ocean sounds are widely available. Others may find specific types of music to be soothing or relaxing. For example, Juan found himself listening frequently to smooth jazz as he struggled to deal with the aftermath of Estelle's assault.

One feature of sound-based relaxation that some people like is that it allows them to focus their attention on something outside of themselves. On the other hand, it can be difficult to employ this type of relaxation when you don't have access to the sound. Imagery-based relaxation is more portable, simply because you can access the image in your mind wherever you might be. The more detailed your mental image, the more you will be able to put yourself into it and relax. And as with the other types of relaxation, the key is practice. The more you do this exercise at home when you are comfortable, the more easily you will be able to picture the scene and the more quickly you can get to it when you are feeling stressed.

Mindfulness and Meditation

Meditation involves the practice of mindfulness, or being present in each moment. Although being mindful can have the effect of relaxing us, that is not necessarily the main goal. Mindfulness entails three skills: focusing your attention on the present moment, adopting an attitude that is free of judgment, and letting go of attempts to control your experiences. Learning to focus attention on the present moment is useful because much of what contributes to our daily stress is thoughts about the past or worries about the future. Focusing on your experience in the moment gives you a reprieve from those sources of stress and thereby promotes relaxation. Similarly, cultivating a nonjudgmental and accepting attitude also can contribute to relaxation. After all, judging ourselves or others contributes to a general sense of dissatisfaction and distress. Suspending judgment of our own thoughts and feelings can decrease how upset we get about the things that our own minds come up with (which can often be worse than what the world hands us!). Mindfulness emphasizes letting go of trying to control things that we cannot control. Instead of our usual efforts to push away unpleasant thoughts and feelings, we practice accepting our thoughts and feelings, just allowing them to be part of our experience. We noted in Chapter 3 that the harder your loved one tries not to think about the trauma, the more she probably thinks about it. Your mind works the same way. Sometimes the harder you try to push things out of your head the more you end up thinking about them.

Mindfulness is not incompatible with any of the other methods of achieving relaxation. In fact, practicing other relaxation methods may enhance your awareness of where you are in the moment and can help you learn to be less judgmental of your sensations, thoughts, and feelings. Likewise, practicing mindfulness skills can enhance other forms of relaxation. However, rather than focusing on achieving relaxation, which can be seen as a form of striving for control, mindfulness emphasizes "letting go" and just noticing (without judging) your experience. Mindfulness programs encourage both formal meditation practice and informal practice of awareness and acceptance in daily life. If you find this focus appealing, you may find it helpful to seek out guidance for mindfulness practice in the form of CDs or practice groups in your area. Resources are listed at the back of the book.

Which One Should You Use?

Research has shown that all of these kinds of relaxation can be helpful for a variety of stress-related problems. We recommend that you try them all to see which methods work best for you. Sometimes the way a person experiences his distress will match up with a particular type of relaxation. For example, Zach noticed that his neck and shoulders often became tense and sore after his brother started trouble at a bar. For Zach, progressive muscle relaxation helped him be aware of the tension and loosen those muscles so that he wouldn't wake up in pain the next day. In contrast, Jenny worried a lot about Marcus, and she found that picturing the beach where they spent their honeymoon comforted her and took her mind away from these worries.

By trying out different techniques, you can find the relaxation technique that works best for you. Joe found that he wasn't very good at picturing a "happy place" in his head, and he thought this sounded kind of silly. But he found that he was really good at focusing his attention on his breathing, and it really calmed him down. Juan, on the other hand, had loved music all his life, and he found that listening to music, or even just thinking about some of the jazz pieces he loved the most, really soothed him. Amanda joined a mindfulness practice group and attended practice sessions weekly. She found this practice helped her quiet her mind at bedtime and maintain her compassion through the stressful times with Paul. As we said earlier, we recommend that you try all of these methods to see what works best for you in which situations. And practice, practice, practice!

Taking Time for Yourself

Even if you eat regularly and get enough sleep, you may be sacrificing other things while trying to care for the trauma survivor in your life. You may be spending time with the trauma survivor at the expense of your own hobbies or interests. You also may be feeling guilty about engaging in enjoyable activities when someone you care about is suffering. Similar to Juan's story at the beginning of the chapter, you might be less engaged in things that you usually find pleasant.

We recommend that you make sure you allow time for things you enjoy or find rewarding. If you're already participating in activities that you enjoy, try to keep them in your schedule, even if you have to spend less time doing them. Juan simply wasn't able to get out and play softball every week, but he worked hard to make every other game that his team played, and he found that the games really relaxed him. He would come home more refreshed, and he felt better able to support Estelle.

You may be devoting so much time and so many resources to the trauma survivor in your life that you can't think of any way you could do something nice for yourself. It can take some effort and creativity, but there is always some way to fit pleasant activities or rewards into your life. After their daughter, Wendy, barely escaped a fire at her apartment, Bill and Mattie cut down their work hours and their recreational activities to take care of her. They had to stop their weekly dinner out, but Mattie made an effort to work the ingredients for one or two enjoyable meals into her weekly grocery shopping. Cooking a favorite meal at home wasn't the same as going out to eat at their favorite restaurant, but Bill and Mattie looked forward to these meals as a break in their busy week.

Social Support

Research has shown that social support tends to ease the effects of stress and helps people recover from a variety of difficulties. One of the best things you can do to help yourself cope with the stress of a trauma survivor in your life is to make use of the social support that you have. Social support usually comes from close friends or family members with whom we can talk about important things. Yousef was extremely worried about his daughter, Marajel, who had been beaten up and mugged in the downtown area of the city where she lived. Yousef had always gotten along with his brother-in-law, Samir, and whenever they got together, he talked about what Marajel was going through and how worried he was about her. Samir sometimes made suggestions about what Marajel could do, but mostly he just listened, and Yousef always felt better after they talked. Sharing the problems you are having with people you feel close to can ease the burden and help you feel less alone.

Sometimes family and friends of trauma survivors can find others who have had or are having similar experiences. Marcus's wife, Jenny, had gotten to know three other women whose husbands were in Marcus's platoon. The women sometimes saw each other during the platoon's deployment, but they found that they got too nervous when they talked too much about where their spouses were. After the soldiers came home, Jenny spent more time with the other three wives. All of their husbands were having problems, some different and some similar, and Jenny found that it really helped her to talk to other people who had an idea of what she was going through. It felt nice to know that she wasn't the only one having those feelings, and after she had lunch with the other wives, she didn't feel as sad or scared.

If you want to talk with someone who is in a similar situation but you don't know anyone personally, you might be able to find a support group in your area. An advantage of support groups is that all the people in the room share in common the situation for which they need support. Diane, whose husband, Roger, served in Vietnam and was still having nightmares about his experiences, didn't know anyone else married to a veteran. When she tried to talk to her sister, Linda, about the difficulties of sharing a bed with him, Linda didn't seem to understand what Diane was so upset about. One day, Diane saw an ad about a VA hospital in her state that provided a support group for wives of combat veterans. She attended, and after a few sessions of listening to others talk about experiences similar to hers, she found the courage to speak up and share some of her own history. She felt welcomed by the group, and she didn't feel so alone. One of the drawbacks of support groups, however, is that, unlike with friends and family, you probably won't know anyone in the group. Many people feel anxious about talking in front of a group or, like Diane, sharing personal information with people they don't know. If you try a support group, we recommend attending for at least several sessions to get a feel for the group and the people in it. If you can't locate a live support group in your area, you might consider joining an Internet-based support group. Numerous such groups exist for all kinds of trauma survivors and their families and loved ones. The Resources section includes a list of organizations and websites that may help you find either live or Web-based support groups.

Maybe you have sources of support in your life but hesitate to burden others with your problems. It's gracious of you to consider others' feelings before you open up to them, but remember that people who care about you usually want to help you, and odds are they will be glad to lend an ear. Joe had always been close to his two younger sisters but didn't feel comfortable talking to them about his struggles with Tom. Then at a family dinner one sister mentioned Tom, and Joe just couldn't keep quiet anymore. He told both of his sisters how much he was struggling with their brother, and he was surprised to find out how supportive and encouraging his sisters were. They never made him feel like he was whining or gossiping, and they told him he could call them whenever he needed to. In fact, one sister said she had no idea why it had taken him so long to talk to them about it!

Treatment

Sometimes the trauma survivor causes so much distress and disruption for the loved ones in her life that social support, relaxation, and good self-care simply are not enough. If you try to get sufficient sleep, eat well, exercise, use social support, and stay engaged in your recreational activities, but still you find yourself feeling sad, anxious, or unmotivated much of the time, you may benefit from treatment yourself. If you've been experiencing many of the warning signs described at the beginning of this chapter for a few weeks or more, we recommend consulting with a medical provider. You may benefit from medication or a brief period of counseling as an additional source of support while you're trying to help the trauma survivor in your life.

The Final Word: Prioritize!

When someone you care about is suffering, it can be very difficult to focus on anything else. The most critical aspect of self-care is prioritizing your own needs. Setting aside time and resources for yourself will enhance your ability to do what you have to do. Remember that if you don't prioritize time for yourself, your needs will take a backseat to all of the stresses and obligations in your life and they will not be met.

As we said earlier in this chapter, it can be a struggle to make decisions that seem to prioritize your own needs above those of someone you care about. As you take time to meet your needs, you may find it helpful to remind yourself that you're taking care of yourself so that you can be there for someone important to you. This won't magically add more time to the day, but it will help you make good decisions for yourself and the trauma survivor in your life. Now, let's talk about how to set your priorities and limits as you try to help your loved one.

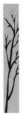

SEVEN

Setting Limits

Marge simply couldn't take it anymore. The shouting, the break-ing things, the punching walls—Walt hadn't hit her yet, but she didn't want to wait until he did. Her mother kept telling her that it's wrong for a woman to abandon her man when he needs her most, that it was her wifely duty to stand by Walt. The way Marge saw it, if he didn't respect her enough to control his temper, he wasn't good enough to be her man.

Even a year later, Graham sometimes felt guilty about leaving Alice. They had been engaged after living together for 3 great years, but then she was raped, and it seemed like everything fell apart. He had resolved to support her through thick and thin, and he did okay for a while, but then things got crazy. She was constantly accusing him of seeing other women, and she had even made harassing phone calls to two female coworkers because she thought he was spending too much time with them. She never left the house, and she got resentful when he did. After coming home a few times to find that she had broken his tools to get back at him for leaving her alone, he had finally had it. He was getting zero respect or love and was sometimes frankly afraid of her. He felt a huge burden had been lifted when he left, but he still wondered whether he had done the right thing.

Jed sometimes wondered if he was doing too much. He had had a hard time when they got back from Kosovo, but after a couple of months things got easier and he readjusted pretty well to the civilian world. Rob seemed to have a lot more trouble. He pretty much never left his parents' house, and the only interaction he had with anyone was playing online war games. In the beginning, if Jed worked hard enough to convince him, Rob would come out. Eventually, Rob just didn't want to do anything, so Jed tried to get other guys from their platoon to visit, even the guys who were out of state. Eventually, Jed would drive over to Rob's parents' place three times a week and spend a few hours with him. It felt weird sometimes, like he was enabling or whatever they called it, and he was giving up a bunch of stuff to spend so much time there, but Rob's parents seemed genuinely thankful for his visits. And besides, you never left a man behind.

Clyde and Nailah had talked about Rob every night before they went to bed. They had suffered through 6 months of his moping and snapping at them. Jed coming over every couple of days was a godsend for them, and they didn't know why he seemed so unaffected by the war while Rob was so clearly hurt. They wondered whether they should continue to let Rob live rent-free, or if throwing him out might force him to make some changes. But they kept coming back to one question: "He's our son—how can we throw him out?"

The family and friends of trauma survivors have many difficult decisions to make. You may be struggling with a number of questions about how you should behave around the trauma survivor or how much you should try to do for her. Some decisions may be about minor aspects of your life, such as "Should I stay home and keep her company, or should I go out with our friends like we had planned?" Or "If we know that she'll probably leave as soon as the party starts, should we even invite her?" However, you also may be asking questions about much larger aspects of your life, such as "He scared me when he punched the wall, but I love him—should I leave him?" Or, as in the case of Clyde and Nailah, "Should we throw him out of the house?" You may wonder whether you're doing too much for the trauma survivor. Hearing catchphrases like "enabling" or "tough love" may lead you to wonder whether it would be best to let her struggle on her own. Conversely, you may feel as though you're not doing enough, and you may second-guess your past decisions. Colin struggled with how much to help his son, Russell, after his return from Afghanistan. Colin felt responsible when, after a year of struggling to keep a job, Russell called him from a homeless shelter. He wondered whether, had he given Russell the money he'd asked for, Russell would have been able to stay in his apartment.

As we discussed in Chapter 6, your desire to help can motivate and energize you to do all you can for the trauma survivor, but it also can put you at risk for exceeding your limits and sacrificing your own well-being. You may believe that if you just work hard enough, do more, or give all you can, you can make your loved one better. Marge knew Walt had difficulties before she married him, but she believed that eventually he would get more comfortable with her and her love would win him over. Over time she started to question those assumptions. No matter what she said or did, Walt always seemed angry. She sometimes thought that the harder she tried, the worse he got. She started to wonder, "Can I change him?"

Many loved ones of trauma survivors find themselves choosing between their own needs and those of the survivor. In this chapter we talk about how to determine how much you're willing to do and where to draw the line. We discuss how to choose where to set your limits so that you maximize your ability to help the trauma survivor without sacrificing your own well-being.

You Can't Change Another Person

Before you decide where to set your limits, it's helpful to know what limits already exist. In other words, we're going to identify your options before we work on choosing one. And one of the first limits that you must accept is that you cannot change another person. No matter what you do or how hard you try, you cannot make another person change something about himself.

As you watch the struggles of the trauma survivor in your life, the answer to her problems may seem perfectly obvious to you. But when you try to communicate a solution, she disagrees with you or appears unable to accept what you see as the plain truth. It seems like the harder you try to make your point, the deeper she digs in against you. Jed constantly reminded Rob of all the things he was missing by staying in the house, and every time he saw Rob, Jed encouraged him to get out, get active, and go do something. Jed presented reason after reason why Rob should leave the house, but no matter what angle he tried, Rob didn't budge an inch. In the beginning, Rob argued back, giving reasons why he was avoiding the outside world. But after a while he simply said "no," and that was that. Jed learned the hard way that if another person has made up his mind to live a certain way, it is very difficult to convince him to change.

When catching the fly with vinegar fails, you might try catching it with honey. Loved ones sometimes offer every conceivable reward for the trauma survivor's efforts to change. Rob's parents tried to give him every reason to find a job or go to school. They offered to give him a car, let him live rent-free, even provide a stipend every month over what the GI Bill provided. But no matter what they dangled in front of him, Rob continued to spend most of his time in his room, and his mood worsened. It was a case of learning that you can lead a horse to water but you can't make it drink.

You can provide incentives, as Clyde and Nailah did for Rob when they offered rewards for going to school, but you cannot make him choose the option you want. Recognizing this will not help the trauma survivor, but it can help you feel less upset and frustrated when your efforts do not succeed.

It's Not Your Fault

As you watch someone close to you struggle with severe problems, you may feel helpless. You may tell yourself, "I should be able to help," or "If I were a better partner/parent/sister/daughter/friend, he wouldn't be having such a hard time." As Juan gradually came to realize that he couldn't make Estelle change, he started to wonder whether he was a good husband. Shouldn't he be able to do something to make sure his wife was okay?

Holding yourself responsible for the well-being of the people you care about is a good thing when there is a problem you can solve. It's a bad thing when the problem is out of your control. When you're feeling bad about your loved one's suffering, remind yourself that it's not your fault. You didn't cause the trauma, and you're not the reason your loved one is having difficulty recovering from it. It also is not your fault that you can't make her change. As Juan came to this realization, he felt as though a burden was lifted from him. He didn't feel better about Estelle's difficulties, but the guilt and frustration he had been feeling lessened dramatically when he let himself off the hook for her problems.

Setting Limits: What Are You Willing to Do? And How Willing Are You to Do It?

Right now you may be thinking, "All right, it's not my fault, and I can't make him change, but should I keep bringing him groceries? Isn't that 'enabling'? And what about the drinking? Should I say anything about his drinking? If I'm all he has, how can I stop being around him?"

When another person behaves in a way that's hard for you to understand, and your efforts to help don't work, you are left with a lot of questions about your relationship. At the end of the day, these questions can be boiled down to two key issues: *How big a part of my life is this person? And what am I willing to do to keep him there?* The more you want to keep the trauma survivor in your life, the more you will be willing to do.

Although these are simple questions, they often are very difficult to answer. These are not questions that we can answer for you—no doctor, expert, or authority can tell you how far you should go to support a person who is important to you. These questions go to the heart of your individual values and goals. We can't answer these questions for you, but we can help you identify the important factors you should consider in your decisions.

How Big a Part of Your Life Is This Person?

By picking up this book, you've already shown that the trauma survivor has a significant role in your life. You are willing to spend time reading this book to get more information and learn ways to help yourself and your loved one. Right now you may believe that you will do anything it takes to support him, and your main goal is to find out how to do that. Or you may not know how much you're willing to do because you're already encountering problems with the amount of help and support you're giving and you want to figure out whether you should draw the line, and how to draw it.

Fortunately, supporting the trauma survivor in your life is not an all-or-nothing decision. There is a wide variety of things you can do to help, ranging from things that are easy to things that can interfere greatly with your life. Setting your limit means figuring out how far on this continuum you're willing to go. There may be some things you're happy to do for the trauma survivor and other things that you simply will not do under any circumstances. For example, Juan might be willing to go to the grocery store at night because Estelle is frightened to be out after dark. But he may feel uncomfortable telling callers that Estelle isn't home when she is but doesn't feel like talking. Lucy may be willing to work longer hours to give Ed more time to recover before he gets a job. But if his war experiences lead him to change his mind about having a family, when he and Lucy previously had agreed to have children, Lucy may choose to leave because she is not willing to make that sacrifice.

How Will Helping Affect You?

You may be unwilling to make a major sacrifice no matter how big a part of your life the trauma survivor is. You may, however, be more willing to comply with requests that would only have a minor effect on your life. Penny and Phil worked in the same part of the city, and Penny had always thought it was wasteful for them to take two cars. After Phil was hit head-on by a drunk driver, he felt uncomfortable driving. It was no problem for Penny to give him a ride each day. His workday ended a little earlier, so Phil was usually waiting for Penny when she came out to the parking lot. Greg and his girlfriend, Jeanette, had been together almost 2 years, and one thing he really liked about their relationship was all the things they did together. After Jeanette was assaulted coming out of a restaurant one night, she no longer was interested in going out. She and Greg spent all their nights at home, watching television or playing games. This was too much for Greg; their relationship no longer was what it had been, and he was not willing to tolerate that.

How Will Helping Affect the Trauma Survivor?

In addition to considering the effects of a particular behavior on you, it sometimes can help to think about the effect that your behavior will have on the trauma survivor. Is he asking you to help him get through something difficult so he can get back to his everyday life? Are you being used as a support, a crutch to lean on as he recovers and learns to walk on his own again? If so, then you may be more willing to help. Phil told Penny that he wanted to start driving again but didn't feel safe doing so alone. So he asked her to let him drive them to his workplace, and then she could take the car back to her office. Penny was very willing to help Phil by doing this, even though it cost her about a half-hour of sleep each morning. Juan, on the other hand, could not see how avoiding talking on the phone would help Estelle's recovery, and he was uncomfortable lying for her, so he was not as willing to do that.

Of course, the difference between what is helpful and what would be counterproductive is not always that clear. Behaviors that look beneficial can in fact be detrimental in the long term. Also, keep in mind that very early in the recovery process a person simply may not be able to tolerate something that seems helpful. After Tom's accident, Joe, following the old adage that you have to "get back on the horse," tried to get him into a car again right away. But Tom's anxiety was so great that he couldn't focus on anything while he was driving, which made it dangerous for him to do so at that time. It may be best to consult a professional health care provider to help determine whether particular activities are appropriate, safe, and beneficial. If your loved one is in treatment and you have contact with her therapist, you can check with him to get the answers to some of these questions. For example, Derrick wanted to help his wife, Emma, recover after the car accident, but she was asking him to do a lot for her, some of which she couldn't do because of her injuries and other things that she was uncomfortable doing. Most notably, she hated driving on the highway. Derrick had heard her therapist talk about confronting fears, so he was not sure how much of the highway driving he should be doing for her. After a month of treatment, Emma told Derrick that her therapist requested that he join them in the next session. During that session the therapist told Derrick that treatment would begin to involve Emma in more activities that made her uncomfortable. Derrick asked whether he should be doing the highway driving for Emma. The therapist told him it was a good question and said that for now Emma would be practicing less scary kinds of driving, but that she would work on reducing her discomfort with highway driving later in therapy. Derrick left the session feeling a little more like he was doing the right thing.

Applying Pro–Con Analysis

Deciding how to respond to the trauma survivor's behavior or requests can be challenging. You need to consider what the trauma survivor means to you, how your behavior will affect your life, and how your behavior might affect the trauma survivor. Putting it all together can be confusing. For example, Estelle often became visibly nervous when she and Juan were out at night. She was calmer when they were at home, but she still wasn't her usual talkative, warm self. And when she was at home, she was much more likely to drink than she would be if they went, say, to a movie. She said drinking calmed her nerves, but Juan didn't see how it could be helpful. Plus, Juan was starting to feel lonely because staying home so much meant they weren't seeing their friends like they used to. Juan knew he loved Estelle very much and wanted to help, but all the different aspects of the situation confused him. Similarly, Maggie and Ian struggled when Tess asked to be picked up from school every weekend so she could study at home, where she felt safe. The drive was close to 3 hours each way, and the cost in gas alone was difficult. And though it seemed to them that it would help Tess feel more comfortable, they didn't think bringing her home every weekend would address the actual problem. Still, she was their daughter, and it was a great struggle for them to say no.

In Chapter 3, we introduced decision (pro–con) analysis, a way to analyze the long-term as well as the often more compelling short-term consequences of different decisions. There, we used it to help you help your loved one think about the change process, but you also can use pro–con analysis to help you make decisions you face with the trauma survivor in your life. It can be particularly effective in helping you set limits on what you're willing to do.

As you complete the decision analysis, keep in mind that we tend to focus on the short-term negative aspects of a choice. Let's say you recently injured your knee. You know that physical therapy can be painful, so, if you considered only the short-term pain, you might decide to skip the therapy. If, however, you also considered what your doctor told you about how physical therapy can improve long-term functioning, you might decide that the positive long-term benefits outweighed the short-term costs. To make decisions that you won't regret, you should consider *all* the consequences in both the short term and the long term. Doing so doesn't mean your decisions are etched in stone, of course. Circumstances change, or you may decide to take a particular route for a finite amount of time and then set a different limit. We further discuss the role of time later in this chapter.

You can use decision analysis to look at questions ranging from whether you want to continue living with the trauma survivor to whether it's worth asking her to do more of the housework. The pro–con form can be used for just about any decision in your life besides those related to the trauma survivor. As you did in Chapter 3, simply list all the positive and negative aspects of each option, in the short term (typically "right now") and the long term (this can range from 2 weeks from now to 20 years from now, depending on the situation). Once you've generated all the short-term and long-term positives and negatives, you can look at the overall results and make your decision. Keep in mind that in complex situations there's usually not a perfect answer; all options will have drawbacks. It sometimes can help first to ask whether you can tolerate the negative aspects of a given option and then consider the long-term consequences of that option. Not all decisions related to the trauma survivor will warrant this level of analysis, but to the extent that you notice uncomfortable feelings about some aspects of the situation, or that it is affecting important areas of your life, it may help to step back and look at things systematically in this way.

We've included two examples to illustrate the process. First, let's look at the form that Clyde and Nailah filled out to help them decide whether they would continue to allow Rob to live with them (shown on page 140). They were keenly aware of the money it would cost in the short term (their grocery and electric bills went up substantially), and they also realized they were helping Rob avoid the world. They guessed, however, that he would not live with them forever, so they didn't see any long-term negative consequences associated with his staying with them. And the short-term and long-term possibilities of their son being homeless were too terrible for Clyde and Nailah to think about. So they chose to allow Rob to stay with them.

Marge's pro–con analysis of whether to stay with Walt is shown on page 141. The main considerations for her were the everyday stress of having Walt in the house and also the practical problems of having to move out and start a new relationship. She was aware both of the potential danger that Walt presented and the possibility that if she stayed with him they could have a wonderful life together. Initially,

Marge decided that she would stick it out with Walt unless he hit her; if that ever happened, she would leave the apartment immediately and never return.

The pro–con analysis is a useful tool for helping you decide how much you're willing to do for the trauma survivor in your life. And it's important to note that you may decide that you are willing to do one thing but not another. For example, Nailah and Clyde may be willing to allow Rob to continue to live with them, but they may draw the line at driving him everywhere. You have the right to look at each decision individually to determine whether it is something you are willing to do.

"Am I Being Selfish?"

You may be reading this and thinking, "How can I say no to him? He fought in a war!" Or maybe, "It's not her fault she was assaulted—am I being selfish?" Remember that you have the right to say no. You have a right to decide what you are and are not willing to do and to choose your behavior accordingly. It sometimes can be difficult to communicate this to someone who wants something from you and is not getting it (we talk about how to communicate your needs next in Chapter 8), but it is still your right.

Wallace struggled with this problem when his wife, Maria, asked him to drive to the other side of town to purchase marijuana for her. Maria had been a medic in Afghanistan for 7 months and was experiencing disturbing memories of things she saw happen to civilians while she was there, things she could not stop. Maria was on edge all the time, and she smoked marijuana most evenings because she said it was the only thing that calmed her. Wallace had to admit that it seemed she was right. On nights when Maria smoked, she snapped at him less and was much less restless in bed. On nights she didn't smoke, she stayed up late, and when she finally came to bed, her sleep was fitful.

Maria was getting increasingly uncomfortable about leaving the house at night and driving, so she had been asking Wallace to do more and more for her. Wallace knew that most people thought marijuana wasn't a "serious" drug like cocaine or heroin, but still it was illegal, and Maria's job as a nurse would be in serious jeopardy if her supervisors found out she was smoking. Wallace didn't feel comfortable telling her she couldn't smoke, but he felt even less comfortable going to an address on the other side of town to buy drugs. Wallace also knew that Maria couldn't rely on marijuana forever; it was helping her sleep but it wasn't solving the problem.

When Wallace started refusing to buy marijuana for Maria, she became angry. She pointed out that Wallace had been willing to take time off from work to take her to meet with a therapist, so why shouldn't he be willing to do this for her? When Wallace told her he wasn't comfortable because it was illegal and it wasn't going to help, Maria accused him of trying to control her behavior.

Is Wallace trying to control Maria's behavior? Or is he controlling her even without trying to? This is a tough question. Wallace is not forcing Maria to do anything, and he's not even telling her what he thinks she should do. He has not forbidden her to smoke, and has not even told her whether he thinks she should smoke. However, he has told her what he will and will not do. Wallace has every right to choose his own behavior, and, if you look closely at this example, this is exactly what he is doing. He has the right to choose how he will respond to Maria. Notice that Maria can still choose to do whatever she wants to, regardless of what Wallace decides.

"How Do I Know I'm Doing the Right Thing?"

Both Maria and Wallace have the right to make their own choices, and we want you to remember that you do too. If you examine the pros and cons thoroughly in both the short term and the long term, you will make the best decision for you and for the trauma survivor in your life. Although decision analysis can help you make a well-informed choice, it does not guarantee that things will turn out the way you expect. The ways that different choices will affect you and your loved one are not always obvious ahead of time. Also, over time, people and circumstances change in ways that often we can't anticipate. The best decision under the current conditions may not be the best decision in 6 weeks or 6 months, under an entirely different set of conditions.

The effects of trauma can wax and wane over time, so we recommend that you periodically reexamine your pro–con analysis to see whether the factors that affected your decision have changed. Your loved one's symptoms may improve or get worse, which may affect your decisions. Marge had initially decided that she would stay with Walt and try to preserve their relationship—unless he hit her. But 4 months after the pro–con analysis, Marge witnessed Walt assault a man in a bar because the man bumped into her by accident. Marge decided then and there that she couldn't feel safe around Walt. She realized that she had underestimated how likely he was to be violent when he was angry, and she did not want to wait until he hit her to leave. Later that week, she moved out.

Also, your ability to help the trauma survivor in your life may change over time. If some of the difficulties associated with supporting him are resolved, you may reevaluate the situation and choose to provide support that you previously had been unable to give. Or the opposite may occur—obstacles may develop that alter your choices. After a few months of struggling with the time and costs of driving Tess home from school every weekend, Ian was laid off from his job. He and Maggie simply no longer could afford the gas costs of driving back and forth to pick up Tess and bring her home. They simply had to stop.

You may have noticed that several of the examples of decision analysis we have described include the possibility that the trauma survivor might get better. For example, Clyde and Nailah's pro–con analysis on page 140 includes long-term considerations like "he won't live here forever" and "he may lose a chance to get better because of us." Clyde and Nailah can't see into the future, so they do not know how things will turn out. When you make a choice based on the hope that someone you care about will get better, you have the right to review that decision over time. We noted earlier that you are the only one who can set your limits. Remember that you do not set them in stone; you have the right to reevaluate your decision to see how well it is working for you. If nothing is changing, or if the anticipated consequences are worse than you had expected, you have the right to change your mind and choose another course of action. Think of Graham's story at the beginning of this chapter. He had resolved to stay with Alice "through thick and thin," but he had thought she would get better and had not realized how bad things could get. When the situation got worse, Graham reexamined the pros and cons and decided that the best thing for him was to leave. He did not want to reach that point, and he did not want things to be that bad for Alice. But they were, and he had the right to change his mind.

Like Clyde, Nailah, Marge, and Graham, you can't see into the future. So all you can do is make the best choice you can now, realizing that you can reconsider if circumstances change in the future. When you make a well-thought-out and informed decision, considering the short-term and long-term consequences of your options, then you can feel comfortable with the choice you make. Focus on your values and what is meaningful to you and choose wisely!

Clyde and Nailah's Pro–Con Analysis of Whether to Allow Rob to Continue to Live with Them

| | Short-term | | Long-term | |
	Pros	Cons	Pros	Cons
Letting Rob stay here	We can try to help him Know that he's okay Safer with us	Losing money He's mean to us He doesn't seem to be getting better We may be helping him stay away from things	We could help him We might be what he needs to get on his feet.	Drain on our finances—but he won't live here forever Emotionally draining if he doesn't get better
Kicking Rob out	It's calmer in the house We can save money We'll sleep better	Feel guilty Don't know where he is He may get worse Worry about him being homeless	Retirement is a little more certain He may be forced to make changes and get better because he has no choice	He may lose a chance to get better because of us He may never get better He might be homeless

Marge's Pro-Con Analysis of Whether to Stay with Walt

		Short-term		Long-term	
		Pros	Cons	Pros	Cons
Staying with Walt		I love him We have a stable home I can try to help him	I'm always on edge I don't sleep well I don't always feel safe around him	Our life has a chance to be "really good" I would know that I "stood by my man"	What if he never gets better? He could assault or even kill me He might not change
Leaving Walt		I'll feel safer and sleep better I'll be calmer around the house, and less worried overall	I'll be lonely It'll hurt a lot I'll have to find a new place and move He will NOT be happy about it	I can get a new start I can find someone who I'm not scared of Emotional stability	I'll never know what we could have been together if I had stayed

EIGHT

Communicating Your Needs

Liz realized that she had only two ways of communicating with her husband, Mickey, who had been a police officer in a tough urban area for 15 years. When he asked her to do something, she either said yes to avoid confrontation or said no and ended up arguing. She knew Mickey had seen a lot of horrible things in his time as a police officer, and she knew these things bothered him a lot. But she still thought their interactions didn't have to be so heated.

Richard tried very hard to be understanding of his partner's situation. After all, he couldn't know what it was like to do the kind of work he did, risking his life to save other people day after day. So most days he tolerated his bad moods without a complaint. If he was unhappy, he never let Tony know; he just kept his thoughts to himself. Sure, he wanted some things to be different between them, but it didn't seem worth bringing them up and risking an argument. Every now and then, however, things would pile up and he would erupt, yelling at Tony for what seemed like no important reason. Afterward he would apologize and feel ashamed of his behavior, but he didn't really know how to stop himself.

Diane tried explaining to her husband, Roger, over breakfast how frustrated she was at having been passed over for promotion at work again. But Roger responded with his usual bossiness, which *in his calmer moments he attributed regretfully to his experiences in Vietnam. Diane had just wanted a sympathetic ear, but Roger rolled his eyes in exasperation as she talked and finally barked out in the middle of her sentence, "Why don't you just quit whining and do what I've been telling you to do over there for years?" It seemed completely reasonable to Diane that she had objected to Roger's tone, but Roger slammed his mug down on the table so hard that coffee splashed all over his newspaper, which he then threw on the floor as he yelled, "If you don't want to hear my advice, I don't know why you even bother to talk to me!" before storming out of the kitchen. Just thinking about their exchange got Diane worked up all over again, and the first thing she did when she got to the hospital was bang on the door of the chief of staff and demand to know why she had been passed over. She was told that there were concerns about her communication style. Nurses working under her had long complained that she was pushy, didn't listen, and often talked over people. When the chief of staff pointed out twice during their conversation that Diane had interrupted him or spoken to him in a harsh and demanding fashion, Diane was shocked. But suddenly she realized that his complaint sounded eerily familiar.*

Family and friends of trauma survivors often feel as though they're walking on eggshells when they interact with the survivor. You may work hard to keep your voice calm to avoid stressing or startling the survivor in your life. You also may notice that it doesn't take much to set off a disagreement, yelling, or a confrontation. You may wish that the withdrawn, isolated trauma survivor in your life would reach out more. But when he does, argument and discord often ensue, and you may find yourself wishing he had stayed wherever he usually hides out. It can seem like you and the trauma survivor have completely forgotten how to talk to each other.

As we've noted several times, it's very hard to make another person change, and that's true for how a person communicates. There are things you can do, however, that can lead to a productive discussion instead of an argument. In this chapter we describe assertiveness, a way of communicating that respects your rights as well as the rights of the other person. Assertive communication gives you the best chance of getting good results in the short term and the long term. Assertiveness isn't a sure thing that will help you in all situations, but it can give you a better chance of achieving what you want with the trauma survivor or, for that matter, with anyone in your life with whom you find yourself in conflict.

Learning to communicate assertively can enhance your life in many ways. It can improve your effectiveness at work, help you meet your needs in your personal relationships, and deepen the intimacy in your closest relationships. Keeping your feelings bottled up is stressful. Expressing your feelings and opinions to others can reduce that stress. And you might discover that other people actually value your thoughts and opinions, respect your preferences, and welcome the opportunity to consider your needs. You may have more input into decisions and gain a greater sense of control in daily life. Also, assertive communication skills have universal applicability. They can be helpful to nearly everyone who has to communicate with others. In our many years of providing clinical services, we have offered only one therapy group that was open to everyone, regardless of whether they were receiving treatment in our clinics for other problems, and that was a group for assertive communication skills. Nearly everyone finds that learning to communicate assertively can be challenging. Our habitual ways of communicating can be hard to change. It can take a lot of practice to get comfortable communicating your needs, preferences, and feelings directly and respectfully. But with practice, assertiveness can become a habit that can make a big difference in your life.

The Two Extremes: Passive and Aggressive

Juan hated seeing Estelle upset, so he tried to give her everything she asked for. If she wanted pasta for dinner, he would agree. If she wanted to stay home, he would agree. When she wanted to rearrange their bedroom so her side of the bed would be away from the door and windows, he agreed. But over time Juan found himself resenting Estelle for all the changes she made. He missed all the things they used to do, and he didn't like their room the way she had arranged it.

Ed yelled a lot and Lucy had always been scared of people yelling at her. As soon as Ed's voice got loud, she would stop talking and just

give in to what he wanted. A few times she had tried to plead her
case, but he would just yell louder, so she learned that the only way
to make the yelling stop was to give in.

As noted in Chapter 2, experiencing irritability and outbursts of
anger is one of the diagnostic criteria for PTSD. In our experience, frequent and intense anger is one of the symptoms that commonly lead
trauma survivors to seek treatment. Anger and aggression are not the
same, however. Anger is an emotion that we feel inside when we think
something is unfair or unjust, or just not going our way. Aggression is
behavior that attacks others verbally or physically. It can range from
yelling, demanding, name-calling, or putdowns to throwing things,
pushing, hitting, punching, or all-out physical fights. There can be
many reasons why trauma survivors act aggressively. Some trauma survivors act aggressively when they feel angry. Sometimes a trauma survivor might resort to aggressive behavior when suddenly frightened or
feeling trapped. The trauma survivor may have learned that aggression
can get him what he wants. Behaving aggressively may lead to others
giving in to his demands, or it may drive others away and help him
avoid trauma reminders.

Many people respond to anger with passive behavior. You may be
overwhelmed by the force of anger coming from the trauma survivor,
and you may give in without expressing your own needs. Or, as in
Juan's case, you may fear that expressing your thoughts will lead the
survivor to become aggressive or withdraw. You may be so concerned
about upsetting her that you never share your opinion or disagree.

Passive behavior consists of giving in to the other person. The
words spoken, body language, and tone of voice all indicate concession
and meekness. The main benefit of passive behavior is that you can
avoid discomfort in the short term. You spare yourself the discomfort
of being shouted at. The main drawback is that you have no opportunity to get your needs met. Indeed, the other person may not even
know what your needs are or that they are being ignored. With passive
behavior, there also is no way to change anything that you're uncomfortable with. Over time the lack of communication can lead to you
and the survivor feeling distant from each other.

Joe had had enough of Tom making plans with him and then can-
celing at the last minute. When he got to Tom's house to pick him

*up for a fishing trip and Tom backed out, Joe blew up. He had taken
a day off from work for the trip and had spent money on equipment
and bait. He yelled at his brother about letting his life slip away
and about being inconsiderate to everyone around him. He ended
his tirade by stomping out and yelling over his shoulder, "From now
on, if you're not intending to do something, don't call me!" Tom felt
guilty for the next 3 days and didn't hear from his brother for the
next week.*

*About a year after the car accident, Noah realized he and his wife
didn't talk anymore. They either yelled or said nothing at all. It
seemed that as soon as one of them opened his or her mouth, a
shouting match started. In the beginning, he had tried, but her
temper was so bad that shouting was the only thing that she listened to. At least it seemed that way, but when Noah really thought
about it, Debbie wasn't really listening at all. Yes, the shouting got
her attention, and at least she stopped when he got louder than she
did, but they still never managed to solve anything. It really did
seem like nonstop yelling.*

When all of your attempts to talk to and reason with someone are
met with shouting and aggression you may be left feeling frustrated
and powerless. While some may back down and become passive in the
face of aggression, others may strike back, fighting fire with fire and
becoming as aggressive as the trauma survivor. When a loved one who
has been traumatized behaves in an aggressive manner, it's easy to fall
into the trap of responding with more aggression. You may be telling
yourself things like "Who does she think she is? She can't talk to me
that way!" Or "I'm not just going to sit here and take that!" So you
shout right back. This engenders a sense of power and control in the
short term, which can feel good to someone who has felt powerless and
out of control. However, in the long term, responding to aggression
with aggression sets both parties up for a pattern of escalating anger
and shouting.

Isolation and withdrawal by the trauma survivor can make the
loved one feel powerless. Joe had repeatedly tried his best to come up
with creative and fun things for him and Tom to do together, but Tom
kept refusing. Joe felt helpless. No matter what he did, Tom kept withdrawing. So Joe increased the intensity and the volume of his state-

ments. He thought that if he simply got louder, it would be harder for Tom to ignore him. Unfortunately, this often can backfire, pushing the trauma survivor further into isolation. And if it does draw a response out of the survivor, that response can be equally aggressive.

Aggression involves disregarding the rights of other people and using intimidation, bullying, or force to get what we want. When we behave aggressively, we make strong verbal statements and offer little chance for negotiation. A person who is acting aggressively often speaks loudly and may not give the other person a chance to offer any input or feedback. He may get very close to the other person and invade her personal space. He may use threatening gestures, such as leaning in, shaking a fist, or pointing a finger. Aggression can feel good, even empowering, in the moment. ("I'm being strong! I'm not taking abuse from anyone!") What most people don't realize is that we often behave aggressively when we feel threatened or powerless, not strong and powerful. This is exemplified by Joe's verbal aggression toward Tom. Joe acted this way when he was feeling helpless and frustrated about their plans being canceled.

The "Third End" of the Continuum: Passive–Aggressive Behavior

Luanne's husband, Marty, had told her countless times not to bother him in his basement. When the door was closed, he didn't want anyone coming in and talking to him. Luanne always nodded and agreed, because she didn't want to get into an argument with Marty—he snapped so easily, which he said was because of the war. But Luanne hated that he could just disappear and leave her with all the responsibility of the house and their children. So over the years she had come up with ways to disturb him without getting him mad at her. For example, their first-floor toilet was always acting up. Luanne knew how to fix it, but instead, she usually called Marty up from his basement to "take a look at it." When he angrily told her she should have done it, she would shrug and say she had already tried and couldn't do it. He would grumble and swear at the toilet but not at her. And while he was upstairs, she would talk to him, ask him to do other things, and even make him a lunch so he would stay longer.

Passive–aggressive behavior is acting aggressively toward a person in a way that makes it hard for them to see our intentions or blame us for the outcome. Someone who is being passive–aggressive may tell a friend she will do something, never really intending to follow through, and then not do it, coming up with an excuse that leaves her blameless. Passive–aggressive people may think, "I really want to tell you this, but that would be difficult or uncomfortable, so I'll tell you something else but then do what I wanted to do in the first place."

The attraction of passive–aggressive behavior is that it allows us to meet our needs and ignore the other person's needs without his knowing. The major drawback is that people often figure out that there is something false about either what the passive–aggressive person is saying or what he's doing. One patient described passive–aggressive behavior by a friend as "smiling while he screwed me." Not surprisingly, passive–aggressive behavior often is damaging to relationships.

The Middle Ground: Assertiveness

Assertiveness combines the most appealing characteristics of passiveness and aggression without their most glaring drawbacks. Unlike the person behaving passively, individuals acting assertively state their needs clearly and do not avoid the reactions of others. Unlike aggression, assertiveness does not disrespect the rights of others and does not seek to get things by intimidation or bullying. Assertiveness means trying to get your needs met while respecting your rights and the rights of the other people involved. **Assertive communication is direct, honest, clear, concise, and respectful.**

But what are these rights we keep talking about? Jakubowski and Lange, in their wonderful book *The Assertive Option: Your Rights and Responsibilities* (Jakubowski & Lange, 1978), list a number of basic rights that all people have (see the box on the facing page). As you review these, notice which ones you put on hold when you interact with the trauma survivor in your life. For example, have you felt guilty saying no because of what the survivor has gone through, and so you agreed to things that you otherwise would not have? Have you refrained from expressing your true feelings so you wouldn't upset the trauma survivor or start an argument? Have you tried to be perfect and never make any mistakes?

Basic Assertive Rights

1. The right to act in ways that promote your dignity and self-respect as long as others' rights are not violated in the process
2. The right to be treated with respect
3. The right to say no and not feel guilty
4. The right to experience and express your feelings
5. The right to take time to slow down and think
6. The right to change your mind
7. The right to ask for what you want
8. The right to do less than you are humanly capable of doing
9. The right to ask for information
10. The right to make mistakes
11. The right to feel good about yourself

Note. From Jakubowski and Lange (1978). Copyright 1978 by Patricia Jakubowski and Arthur L. Lange. Reprinted by permission of Research Press.

Assertiveness emphasizes your basic rights as a human being. This includes your rights to express your needs, to be heard, and to be treated with respect. Assertiveness also can be more effective in the long term than aggression and passivity. Although assertiveness does not guarantee that you'll get what you want, it gives you much more of a chance than passive behavior. And although in some cases aggression works in the short term, bullying others damages relationships in the long term. Assertiveness, in contrast, can strengthen relationships by respecting the needs of all the people involved.

Is Something Keeping You from Believing You Have a Right to Be Assertive?

For most of us, assertiveness doesn't come naturally. Many people have difficulty being assertive, whether or not they or someone they care about has been traumatized. From early childhood, we are bombarded with messages about how we should treat others and what it means about us if we ask for something or assert our rights. If you notice yourself feeling uncomfortable at the thought of asking for what you want in a direct, straightforward way, then it may help to notice what you are saying to yourself as you contemplate being assertive.

You may notice that you think being assertive sounds a little too aggressive for your taste. Sometimes people confuse assertion with aggression. They think that standing up for themselves inevitably means steamrolling over others, and they see advocating for their own needs as being selfish and uncaring. For example, Richard had trouble being assertive with Tony because Richard had watched his mother ignore her own needs and constantly dote on his father. As a result, he believed that it is selfish to ask for what he wants in a relationship and that focusing on taking care of the other person's needs ensures that he will be loved. Richard tended to think of assertion as aggression, and the last thing he wanted was to be seen as demanding or aggressive. He feared that if he asked for what he wanted Tony would consider him "pushy," and that might drive Tony away.

You also may find yourself thinking that acting assertively is being "selfish." You may believe that being assertive means you are placing your needs above someone else's and that this is wrong. This may be especially difficult when you are thinking about the trauma survivor. You may think that putting aside your needs and deferring to his is the right thing to do. You may tell yourself that doing anything else is self-centered and disrespectful to him. Liz knew that Mickey worked hard, and she felt that he deserved to have a peaceful home. Asserting her own needs seemed selfish, like she wasn't taking his efforts into account. What Liz had a hard time understanding is that assertiveness means valuing both partners' rights, not putting one person over another. She did not have the right to ignore Mickey's needs, but she did have the right to have her own needs respected.

Liz also realized that she was affected by another belief that many women have instilled into them by a male-dominated society: she thought that if she spoke up and asserted herself she was being a "bitch" whom no one would like. When she identified this belief, she tried to think about other people she knew, women and men, who she thought treated other people poorly. She compared their behavior to what she would sound like if she asserted herself by asking Mickey to change his behavior. Liz realized that she had been confusing assertiveness with being mean or a "bitch." She realized that the label "bitch" was a way to judge women when they stood up for themselves. When she actually looked at what she was asking Mickey to change, she realized she was being completely consistent with her assertive rights.

You also may find that you have beliefs about what it means to give up being aggressive. Diane had spent many years dealing with Roger's aggression, and over time she found that the only way she ever felt like she had any control was when she responded with aggression and tried not to let Roger "win." So Diane developed the belief that she had to be aggressive to get her own needs met, and that if she was not aggressive the other person would take advantage of her and disregard her. Feedback she received at work about how she treated others helped her understand that she would not sacrifice any power by allowing others' needs to get met along with her own.

Many of the misconceptions and erroneous beliefs that interfere with being assertive presume that one person's rights are not as important as the other's. Passive people tend to value and respect other people's feelings, opinions, and needs more than their own. Aggressive people tend to put their needs above those of others. The challenge is to value both equally. Finding balance is especially hard when there are good reasons to put the trauma survivor's needs ahead of your own. On top of his preexisting ideas about how to behave in a relationship, Richard thought that Tony was more deserving of respect than he was because of the brave work that he did every day. As a result, Richard had a habit of thinking that Tony's needs were more important than his own, which usually led him to keep his needs to himself. For Richard, learning to communicate assertively was not just about learning how to say what he was feeling and express what he needed, but also learning to believe that his feelings and needs were as important as Tony's. The surprise for him was to learn that Tony thought so too. Tony found it much easier to get along with Richard when Richard was clear about his needs and preferences. Richard was surprised to learn how much of a relief it was for Tony when he didn't have to guess what Richard wanted.

If you think preconceived notions or judgments are keeping you from believing you deserve to be assertive, revisit the Basic Assertive Rights listed on page 149. Also, we have included a list of some of the common preconceptions that interfere with assertiveness on page 152. Examine the list and also take stock of what goes through your mind when you think about being assertive. We have included more balanced alternate beliefs that you can use to combat what your mind tells you so that you can be more assertive. If these counterarguments and reminders of your rights are not enough to galvanize your efforts to be assertive, it might help to speak to a counselor or other mental health professional.

Common Self-Statements That Interfere with Assertiveness

Self-statement	Assertive right being ignored	New self-statement
If I don't think of others before myself, I'm being selfish.	The right to act in ways that promote your dignity and self-respect as long as others' rights are not violated in the process.	Putting my needs above someone else's would be selfish. But, my needs are as important as others' and I have the right to have my needs respected.
Assertiveness means thinking I'm better than other people.	The right to ask for what you want.	My needs are not any more important than anyone else's, but they also are not less important.
[for women] Asking others to change makes me a bitch.	The right to be treated with respect.	No one has the right to be mean to other people or mistreat or disrespect them, but I do have the right to have my own needs met while respecting the needs of others.
Giving in to other people means they win and I lose.	The right to act in ways that promote your dignity and self-respect as long as others' rights are not violated in the process.	One person getting his needs met does not mean that the other person does not. Through negotiation and compromise, we both can get needs met and "win."

If I tell people what I don't like about them, it will hurt their feelings and make me a bad person.	The right to experience and express your feelings.	If someone is behaving in a way that violates my rights, I have the right to tell him that. It may hurt his feelings, but that is not my intention. I have the right to feel the way I feel.
I should always help other people. It is good and right to put others' needs ahead of my own.	The right to do less than you are humanly capable of doing; the right to say no and not feel guilty.	It is good to help other people, but I have the right to act in a way that gets my needs met. I have the right to give my own needs equal priority with others' needs.

How to Be Assertive

Although it may feel awkward at first, with practice you can learn to feel more comfortable communicating assertively. Below is a set of basic steps for being more assertive. Master these and you will be well on your way to improving the quality of your interactions with your loved one.

Say Clearly What Is Bothering You

Assertive communication is honest. If the trauma survivor in your life is acting in a way that hurts you, tell her that. Do so in a clear, concise, direct manner. First, make sure to be *specific* when explaining what bothers you, and try to avoid generalizations. Joe wanted to convey to Tom why he was angry with him. Telling Tom that "It's frustrating to me when you keep backing out of the plans we make" is much clearer than a global put-down like "You're a lousy brother." Well-defined behaviors are much easier to adopt than fuzzy ones. For Tom, it would be hard to know where to start if he were being asked to be "less lousy as a brother," as opposed to Joe asking that he back out of plans less often. Second, be direct and concise. Don't dance around the issue. Note that Joe's statement above gets right to the point. In contrast, the following statement is reasonably clear but not direct: "Ever since your accident it seems like you don't know what you want anymore. You make plans and then change your mind so often it makes my head spin. I am tired of your wishy-washiness. One of these days I hope you figure out what you want and let me know. You need to just learn how to stick with a plan for once!"

Tell the Other Person How His Behavior Affects You

After you state the specific behavior that bothers you, tell the other person exactly *why* it bothers you. As with the description of the behavior, try to avoid general remarks like "That's just wrong" or "That's not what a wife should do." Instead, state specifically how you are affected by the trauma survivor's behavior. For example, Luanne might say to Marty, "When you spend all your time in the basement and don't share in the household activities, I feel like I'm running the house alone, and that hurts me." Similarly, after telling Tom that he keeps backing out of their plans, Joe might say, "When I take time off from work and you cancel our plans, I lose the time and money I'd earn. It seems like you don't care about me, and that hurts." When discussing how you feel about the survivor's behavior, take ownership of your own feelings rather than blaming him. Say, for example, "I was annoyed that you left and I had to do all the work myself" rather than "You make me so angry when you just leave in the middle of everything."

State What You Would Like to Be Changed

Assertive behavior involves not only expressing how the other person's behavior affects you but also how you would like things to be. Often, we fall into the trap of assuming that other people can read our minds. Juan, for example, often found himself thinking, "We're a married couple. She must realize that we don't ever go anywhere. Why would she be okay with that?" He always went along with what Estelle wanted and then was surprised when she never volunteered to go along with what he wanted to do. Estelle, meanwhile, was making her choices out of fear, with the goal of avoiding anything that felt uncomfortable or dangerous. She assumed Juan was okay with that *because he never told her otherwise.*

Juan decided to assert his own needs and let Estelle know how her insistence on staying home and not socializing was affecting him. He told her that when they stayed home every weekend and skipped getting together with their friends he felt lonely, isolated, and trapped. Next, he told Estelle what he would like. He said, "I would like us to go out of the apartment at least some of the time," and, "A couple of nights during the week I would like to go out and spend some time with my friends." Being specific about what you want gives the other person an opportunity to reconcile that with what she wants. As with Richard and Tony earlier in the chapter, it relieves the other person of trying to read your mind.

Offer Compromise or Describe the Consequences

A good rule of thumb when expressing your needs is to be flexible in asking for change. Note that Juan said he would like to go out "at least some of the time." He was not demanding that Estelle do things entirely his way, but he was asking for a compromise. He also suggested another compromise: that he sometimes go out without her. Approaching the other person with a willingness to meet her halfway will open the door for negotiating a solution that meets both of your needs.

Another useful strategy is to let the survivor know how the requested change would help you. Juan told Estelle that he would be happier if there were more people in his life. Lucy told Ed that she would feel safer and more comfortable in her own home if he yelled at her less. Both Estelle and Ed cared about their partners. When they heard that change on their part would be beneficial to their partners, they felt less defensive and were able to understand why they were being asked to do things differently.

You have the right to ask for what you want, so you don't have to offer something in exchange for it. But your willingness to concede something the other person wants might make him more likely to make the change you're requesting. Luanne might tell Marty that if he spends the morning with her he can have the afternoons to himself. Similarly, Joe could give Tom a deadline for canceling plans, such as three days ahead. If Tom canceled by then, Joe would have time to reschedule the time off; if Tom didn't cancel that far ahead, Joe would expect him to follow through on the plans.

Steps for Communicating Assertively

1. Say clearly what is bothering you.
2. Tell the other person how his behavior affects you.
3. State what you would like to be changed.
4. Offer compromise or describe the consequences.

Other Tips for Being Assertive

• *If you are assertive and you are met with aggression, maintain a direct, straightforward, nonattacking tone.* Noah knew that he and Debbie quickly escalated to the point where they were shouting at each other. When this pattern is in place, assertiveness is often met with aggression, even if the person being assertive is following all the rules explained here. It's important to remember that someone who is used to reacting this way can be expected to continue to react this way. Don't get drawn into the aggressive pattern of interacting.

• *If the other person reacts to your request for change with a complaint of his own, acknowledge his issue and then restate your initial point.* When others give us negative feedback, our first instinct is to strike back at them. So your assertive request for a change may be met with criticism. For example, when Noah told Debbie that her tendency to snap at him when he asked her to do something was making him uncomfortable, she immediately replied, "Oh yeah? Well I'm sick of you always criticizing me!" This is the sort of global, nonspecific remark that can turn a productive conversation into an argument. For example, if Noah responded with "Oh no, I'm not!" or "That's because you're always screwing up!" then the interaction would be likely to escalate in aggressive exchanges from there. The opportunity to resolve his original concern might be lost and his chances of getting his needs met would diminish.

To avoid being sidetracked, it's critical to stay focused on the issue at hand. Sometimes this can be as easy as repeating yourself. If Noah responded to Debbie's attacks on him with some variation of "When you snap at me when I ask you to do things, it sounds like you don't care about my needs and I feel hurt," eventually Debbie may run out of attacks and Noah will still be set on the same message. Often it helps to acknowledge your partner's complaint. Noah might say, "Okay, so you think I'm too critical. I'm willing to discuss that, but first I want us to discuss the way I feel when you snap at me."

• *If you know that bringing up a certain topic will make the trauma survivor angry, plan and rehearse what you want to say.* It can sometimes be difficult in the moment to react in an assertive way when the other person begins shouting. You can plan ahead of the talk what you want to say and how best to say it in a nonthreatening way. In fact, you also may be able to anticipate what the other person will likely say back, and then you can plan your response to that. For example, Joe knew if he told Tom that "When we make plans and then you cancel at the last minute, it hurts me, and it affects me at my work," Tom would probably initially reply with something like "Well, I'm not asking you to make plans or do things; you could just leave me alone." Joe spent some time figuring out how to respond to this before he brought the topic up with Tom.

How Do You Know Whether Assertiveness Is Working?

There are a variety of ways that assertiveness can lead to positive changes in your interactions with others, including the trauma survivor in your life. The most obvious is that you will have a better chance of getting your needs met. Joe felt uncomfortable bringing up the topic of Tom's backing out of their plans, but he kept reminding himself that it was really bothering him, so he finally did. He felt even worse as he watched Tom visibly squirming, and for the first time he saw that Tom was aware of how he was affecting others. He talked about how sometimes he got so anxious that he just couldn't leave the house, but in the end he accepted Joe's compromise about a deadline for canceling. As Joe drove home that day, he felt hopeful that things might be better with his brother.

Assertiveness also can improve the quality of your interactions with the trauma survivor, even if you don't get what you want any more of the time. Liz made a commitment to herself to be more assertive with Mickey whenever they made decisions, and at first it wasn't easy. It seemed like the more she tried to be calm and assertive, the more aggressive he got. But over time she noticed that his aggressiveness decreased, and he started to behave more assertively toward her. He didn't give in to her requests any more than he had, but her reluctance to bring anything up with him decreased dramatically. She felt more like he was actually listening to her and more like she had the right to ask for what she wanted.

Keep in mind that assertiveness won't always change the other person, but if you stick to it, you may feel better about yourself. By telling Tony more clearly what he wanted, Richard didn't always get his needs met, but he felt a more equal balance of power in their relationship. Although his assertiveness led to more disagreements than when he was passive, Richard was proud that he had become more direct and honest in his interactions with his partner.

What If Assertiveness Doesn't Work?

Assertiveness will increase your chances of getting your needs met and improving the relationship but it does not guarantee this will happen. The other person may resist your efforts to communicate in an assertive, constructive way. As we noted in Chapter 2, this probably is not personal—it may reflect general interpersonal difficulties. The trauma survivor likely is not trying to push you out of her life. Rather, she may be afraid of being close to you. Trauma survivors often have difficulty trusting others. They may be afraid of being vulnerable or believe that others will judge them. The survivor in your life may be trying anything she can to keep her distance. Ed had used anger for many years to keep Lucy away from him. He had lost people close to him in Afghanistan, and he did not want to feel that kind of hurt again. Although he knew that he would do anything for Lucy, he was scared of loving her, because then he could be hurt. When she told him that she would feel safer if he didn't yell at her as much, he felt terrible that he had scared her, but part of him also was scared of getting closer to her. It made him feel vulnerable and helpless. Alternately, the trauma survivor may have so much difficulty experiencing his own emotions that his anger escalates out of control too quickly for him to do anything about it. He may be afraid of lashing out in anger, so he remains detached from you in effort to keep this from happening.

Many people don't recognize differences between styles of communicating. Some people who are aggressive do not realize that the way they communicate is off-putting. They may think that they need to be firm and forceful to get their needs met, and they may confuse this with being assertive. Diane was surprised to hear that her communication was perceived as aggressive. She thought it was necessary to be firm and directive with the staff in order to be respected and get things done. It was never her intention to be pushy. In her effort to be an effective leader, she ended up adapting the style Roger had used with her and the kids, if for no other reason than that she had seen it efficiently head off long debate. Of course, when she stopped to think about it she realized that this style had strained Roger's relationships with many people. Peers obviously didn't like his attempts to dominate them and force his decisions on them, and the kids were sometimes afraid of their own father. Diane wanted people to respect her and follow her instructions, and she wanted to be an effective decision maker and efficient supervisor, but she didn't want people to be afraid of her. She committed herself to learning a calm and pleasant yet businesslike way of communicating with her staff. As she made these changes, she began to see that when her style of communication demonstrated her respect for others, they respected her more. As a result, she actually became more effective at her job. She also carried this into her relationship with Roger. Whereas previously she had felt the only way to get him to listen to her was to yell back, now she found that when she spoke calmly, he calmed down too.

It's important to remember that assertiveness can take time and practice. Just because the first time you try to be assertive you end up in an argument does not mean that you will fail the second time you try, or the fifth, or the twelfth. Noah noticed that the first few times he tried assertiveness with Debbie she blew up at him even more than usual. She was getting even angrier because he *wouldn't* fall into the familiar pattern of arguing. But then, he noticed that after a few minutes of shouting without him shouting back her tone gradually softened. Eventually, Debbie would yell once or twice and then take a deep breath and respond to what Noah was saying. If Noah had abandoned the effort early on, he never would have seen the results. So if you want to experience the benefits of assertive communication in your relationships, our advice to you again is: Don't give up!

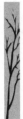

PART III

Coping with Specific Traumas

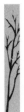

NINE

When Someone You Love Has Been Sexually Assaulted

Please be warned that the following material is explicit, and some readers may find it uncomfortable to read. We can't help you understand the phenomenon of sexual assault without being clear about what we are talking about. If you find the explicit descriptions intolerable, you may choose to skip this chapter. If your loved one survived a sexual assault, however, you will probably find the information valuable. Your discomfort may diminish as you proceed, and becoming more comfortable with these issues may make it easier for you to be supportive to your loved one.

Estelle was on her way home after a late night at the office. She had walked that street many times before, at all hours, without incident. Nothing seemed any different that night. She was just nearing the entrance to the subway station when the men appeared, seemingly out of nowhere. At first she thought they were asking her for directions, so she was friendly to them. But then she realized they were grabbing at her and saying vulgar things, so she tried to go around them and make her way to the station. But they followed her, and when they grabbed her and pulled her toward the alley she realized how strong they were, and suddenly she became terrified. As they dragged her she started to scream and punch at them. But late as it was, no one was around to hear her screams. Besides, one of them held his large hand over her mouth, so she could hardly breathe. Her struggles were useless against their tight grip, and after a while she just lay still. One of them was holding her and saying horrible sexual things in her ear with alcohol strong on his breath while the other pulled his pants down and pulled out his penis as he yanked at her skirt. She was horrified and disgusted at the same time and felt utterly helpless. Then, just as he came closer to her, a car door slammed in the street and startled them. The man holding her loosened his grip for a moment, just long enough for her to free herself. She sprung up with more energy than she had ever felt in her life. She swung her purse at one assailant's face and kicked the other in his shin. She fled to the station, down the stairs and boarded the next train home. When she walked in the door disheveled and broke down in tears Juan was horrified and insisted they call the police.

Tess was a sophomore in college and a dedicated student who spent most nights studying. She occasionally went out with friends for pizza or movies, but she wasn't much into drinking and had never experimented with drugs—she just didn't see the point. But after almost 2 years at college, she realized that her social life was lack- ing—she'd been on only a few dates and still had never had a boyfriend. So when her friend Ariel suggested they check out the party at the frat house, she decided maybe it was time to see what she was missing. Besides, her friend pointed out that the guys in that fraternity were really hot—maybe she would meet someone she liked. So she went out of her way to put on a cute outfit and paid more attention to her makeup and hair than she usually did. When they arrived, the party was well under way and a lot of the other kids were drinking beer, so even though she wasn't much of a drinker, Tess thought she should have one to fit in. She spotted Tommy from her chemistry class across the room and smiled at him. A little while later he came over and started talking to her and then asked her to dance. She danced, then had a few more beers, and soon she was talking to his friend Campbell, who she thought was pretty good-looking. He seemed interested in her, so when he suggested she try a shot of hard liquor, she figured "Why not?" She was having a good time, and she was afraid to spoil it by not going along with them. After a few shots she felt kind of woozy, so when they led her toward the couch in a back room to sit down it seemed like a good idea. At first they were just talking and drinking more, but then she started to realize it was getting late and she wondered where Ariel was. When she got up and headed toward the door, Tommy led her back to the sofa and told her that her friend was dancing and having a good time like her, so she should just relax. By now, her head was spinning, so sitting down again seemed the easiest thing to do. But she started to feel uncomfortable when she realized he was pulling her shirt up, and when she asked him to stop, he didn't. Next thing she knew they were both groping her all over, and she got up and went for the door again. But when she opened the door, another guy she didn't know pushed her back into the room and locked the door behind him. Realizing she was trapped, she suddenly was terrified. She screamed, but realized no one could hear her over the loud music.

Jake had been spending weekends at his uncle Harry's house for a couple of years after his father left the family. One day when he was 6, his uncle took him on his lap, playing "horsey," and then slowed down, and as he did, his hand went down between Jake's legs and started rubbing him there and telling him how much he liked him. Jake was confused. His mother was always telling him not to touch himself—what was his uncle doing? Then Harry set Jake next to him, opened his own fly, and took his penis out of his pants. Jake was shocked—he had never seen anyone's wiener but his own. He placed Jake's hand on it and told him, "Be a good boy and pet it, just like you pet your hamster." Jake felt really uncomfortable, and he thought that something must be wrong here, but his uncle was a grown-up, and his mom always told him that when he was there his uncle was in charge, so Jake did as he was told, even though it didn't feel at all like his hamster. It got bigger, and his uncle started making funny sounds and didn't seem at all like himself, and then sticky gooey stuff squirted everywhere, and his uncle smiled, patted him on the head, and told him what a good boy he was. Afterward, Uncle Harry told him that he couldn't tell anyone or his mother would never let him come home. This made no sense—if he was a good boy, why did he have to keep it secret? Every weekend after that, even as his uncle made Jake do more and more icky things, Jake kept waiting for his mother to find out what was going on and rescue him, but she never did.

Among various types of trauma, interpersonal assaults such as sexual assault and sexual abuse are associated with the highest risk for developing PTSD. Sexual assaults and abuse frequently involve both a physical violation of the body and a violation of personal trust. Survivors of sexual assault and abuse are at risk for a range of problems, such as depression, anxiety, substance abuse, eating disorders, dissociative disorders, and problems with interpersonal relationships. The pervasive effects of sexual abuse and assault on survivors' emotional well-being and daily life often last for years and even decades beyond the events. You might be aware that your loved one survived sexual abuse or assault early in life, like Jake, or more recently, like Estelle. Either way, you probably feel somewhat helpless—powerless to have protected the person you care about from the assault and to soothe the person's pain now. You may feel confused by some of the changes you've seen in your loved one or wonder how abuse from long ago has been shaping the behavior of someone you love. In this chapter we discuss how sexual assault and abuse can affect the survivor and his relationship with you. Understanding the common ways that sexual assault can affect your loved one will help you be better able to cope with these effects on your lives and provide critical support during the healing process.

How Is Sexual Abuse Different from Sexual Assault?

To be perfectly clear, we want to define our terms. We'll explain what we mean by *sexual assault, sexual abuse,* and also *sexual harassment,* another experience that can sometimes be traumatic.

Sexual Assault

When we speak of sexual assault, we mean being forced or coerced to have sexual contact against your will. This includes contact imposed on a person who is intoxicated or impaired by drugs. Although most perpetrators are men and most victims are women, sexual assault can happen at any age to a person of any gender or sexual orientation. The sexual contact might involve sexual intercourse, as when the term *rape* is applied, but it also can include many other forms of sexual contact. A person might be forced to engage in anal sex or oral sex, or she may be penetrated with a hand or object. Sexual assault can include unwanted fondling, groping, grabbing, or disrobing of the victim or forcing the victim to touch the perpetrator's genitals or perform sexual acts on the perpetrator. The sexual acts may occur through use of physical force or captivity or by threats of harm, including with a weapon such as a gun or knife. As we talk about later, the victim may or may not fight back, and even an "attempted" assault can be traumatic. When we think of sexual assaults, we usually think of a woman being assaulted by complete strangers, such as what Estelle experienced. Most sexual assaults, however, are perpetrated by a person known to the victim; fewer than 20% are perpetrated by strangers.

Sexual Abuse

When we talk about sexual abuse, we are referring to unwanted sexual contact experienced by a person usually under the age of 16, although persons of diminished mental capacity, such as those with a developmental disability, also can be sexually abused. Typically, the perpetrator is known to the victim and usually is older than the victim, thereby in a position of relative power. Often the sexual contact is forced or coerced, but in many cases a victim below the age of consent may have complied out of fear, confusion, or shame. The sexual contact may have involved vaginal, oral, or anal penetration, or it might have been limited to touching or kissing the victim in sexual ways or having the victim touch the perpetrator. In some instances the victim might not have been touched but was subjected to visual inspection or made to view pornography or watch others perform sexual acts. When sexual abuse occurs at a young age, the victims may not recognize the experience as a violation until many years later.

Perpetrators of sexual abuse can include family members or relatives, neighbors, family friends, clergy, teachers, scout masters, babysitters, caretakers, or anyone who might have contact with the minor. Although many perpetrators are male, women also sometimes sexually abuse children or adolescents. Often such persons coerce the sexual contact by using their position of power over the child, such as the priest who molested John when he was in the church choir at age 12. Sometimes the abuser threatens to harm the victim or his family members if he doesn't go along with the sexual behavior or if he tells anyone what happened. Jake felt uncomfortable and frightened when his uncle touched him the first time. At first his uncle told him that if he told his mother about it she wouldn't let him come home; then he told Jake that if he told others they too would reject him and would not believe him. Later, his uncle also threatened to hurt Jake's younger brother if he told anyone. Jake kept quiet for many years out of shame and fear. Often there are multiple episodes of sexual abuse by the same perpetrator over a period of months or years. Also, some victims experience abuse by multiple perpetrators—this might happen because the primary caretaker is unavailable or unable to protect the child or is inaccessible or unresponsive when the child reports the abuse. Sometimes the survivor of sexual abuse never discloses the abuse to anyone.

Sexual Harassment

Sexual harassment refers to a wide range of situations, often in a workplace or educational setting, in which a person is subjected to unwelcome sexual advances that can take the form of intimidation, bullying, coercion, or force. The behaviors can range from mild transgressions and annoyances to actual sexual abuse or assault when the victim is forced, pressured, or manipulated into engaging in unwanted sexual contact. Usually, although not always, the perpetrator is a person in authority who wields some form of power over the victim. The perpetrator may make direct or implicit threats to harm the victim in financial or other ways, such as getting the victim fired, withholding a promotion, or lowering academic grades. The lines between harassment and assault sometimes can be blurred. Vanessa was a rookie in the police force when her sergeant approached her in the locker room, pushing her up against the lockers and groping her breasts. When she protested, he reminded her that he got to decide whether she would be promoted or even keep her job. She had always dreamed of becoming a detective and had worked hard to get into and graduate from the police academy. She was afraid all her hard work would be for nothing if she went against his wishes, so she let him touch her. This happened on a daily basis for a while until one day the sergeant followed her to her car after work and insisted she let him in. She was scared to say no, so she did. When he insisted she perform oral sex on him, she didn't want to, but she worried that if she lost her job she would lose the career for which she had worked so hard. Besides, he had a gun on his belt, and when she hesitated he pointed to it, so she went along with his request.

Not all sexual harassment involves coerced sexual contact. Various offensive behaviors, such as stories or jokes about sex, conversation about sexual topics, or unwanted sexual advances can create a hostile work environment and constitute sexual harassment. Although it is less likely to result in PTSD, there are mental health consequences of this type of sexual harassment as well. Sexual harassment is a form of illegal employment discrimination in many countries, so sometimes the victim may be involved in legal proceedings related to the experiences, which can be very stressful. Sexual harassment that includes sexual assault is most likely to have the kind of lasting effects that we describe below.

How Common Are Sexual Assault and Abuse?

Your loved one is not alone. Approximately one in four women and one out of eight men in the United States have experienced a sexual assault at some point. Estimates are that 10–15% of men and 20–30% of women have experienced some form of sexual abuse as a child. Most of the statistics on the frequency of sexual assault and sexual abuse are based on surveys. Experts in the field generally believe that many survivors of sexual assault or abuse are not willing to disclose their experiences, so these figures likely underestimate the scope of the problem.

Unwillingness to disclose a history of sexual abuse or sexual assault is not limited to surveys. It's important to realize that, due to the shame and stigma around sexual assault, many survivors of sexual assault and abuse never report the experiences to anyone. As a result, they often *feel* alone. You may find that reassuring your loved one that she is *not* alone can go a long way toward reducing that sense of isolation and starting her on a path to healing.

How Do Sexual Assaults Affect Survivors?

Among various types of trauma, sexual assaults are particularly devastating to a survivor's sense of emotional well-being. Estimates are that 30–65% of sexual assault survivors develop PTSD and 30–40% suffer from clinical depression. Sexual assaults affect the survivors' sense of safety and comfort in the world, ability to trust others, trust in their own judgment, and feelings of competence and self-worth. Survivors of sexual assault and abuse are at risk for a range of mental and physical health problems.

Fear and Anxiety and PTSD

If your loved one was sexually assaulted, she experienced a fundamental violation of her sense of safety in the world. She is vulnerable to fear and anxiety as well as the reexperiencing, avoidance, and hyperarousal symptoms of PTSD. As discussed earlier, these are normal reactions to trauma that are often present in the initial period following the event. Approximately 95% of sexual assault survivors experience reexperiencing, avoidance, and hyperarousal symptoms in the 2 weeks immediately following the trauma. Three months later about 50% of women still experience symptoms, which is a high percentage compared to many other types of trauma (Rothbaum et al., 2006). The National Women's Study reported that almost one-third of all rape victims develop PTSD sometime during their lives, and 12% of rape victims suffer from the disorder at any given time (Resnick et al., 1993).

PTSD is especially likely when the victim was extremely frightened or felt helpless or powerless during the assault, which is often the case when there was vaginal, anal, or oral penetration and when physical force, restraint, or a weapon was involved. When Sinead was raped, her assailant, a large man with a bushy beard, held a knife to her throat and told her that if she disobeyed a single order from him he would gut her like a fish. Sinead was so frightened that she could barely think, so she made sure to do exactly what he asked, even though she felt revulsion. Afterward, she was terrified whenever she left the house and had a hard time relaxing even at home. She had nightmares about the assault and became very upset whenever she saw a man with a beard, even on television. Whenever she encountered someone wearing the cologne her rapist wore, she felt nauseated, weak, and trembled inside.

Problems with guilt, shame, or anger, or complications such as injuries and scars, can exacerbate PTSD. At first Juan didn't understand—Estelle fought back and got away from the men, so he thought she should feel good that she was able to protect herself. As time went on, however, he learned more about the details of what happened. He came to realize that even though nothing bad had ever happened to Estelle before, she had always thought of herself as a "streetwise" person who was alert to her surroundings and protective of herself. She was caught off guard by the assailants, and as a result she no longer trusted her own judgment about safety when she left their apartment. He began to see that even though she had escaped, she had felt really scared and helpless when they held her down before she was able to fight them off. Estelle's therapist explained that the intense fear and helplessness had triggered her fight–flight response in a big way. Estelle was mortified, realizing that for a few moments she completely froze and stopped fighting back. She couldn't make sense of this and thought that it meant that in some way she had participated in the assault. She was confused and embarrassed to tell Juan about this.

Estelle was able to resolve her distress about this when her therapist informed her that freezing is a third element of the fight–flight response that kicks in when a person is helpless to flee or fight back. She was enormously relieved when he pointed out that this is an involuntary reaction that did not mean she wanted to be raped. Juan also had noticed that Estelle was preoccupied with trying to figure out how she could have prevented it from happening, even though from his point of view there wasn't really much she could have done. During her therapy, Estelle also came to see that her options that night were pretty limited and she had no reason to anticipate the assault.

Depression and Low Self-Esteem

About a third of rape survivors will experience depression at some time in their lives. After the assault, Estelle withdrew from friends and family and many of the activities she used to enjoy. Juan was frustrated that over time she seemed less and less interested in doing anything. Sometimes they ended up arguing when he tried to get her to go out with him. Why couldn't she see that everything was okay and she could get back to her life? He didn't know what to do to cheer her up. She even seemed to be losing weight, and she was grumpy in the mornings when she woke up too early.

Depression also is common among those who experienced sexual abuse in childhood. This may be due to the fact that childhood sexual abuse often occurs in the context of an unsupportive family with many life problems. Jake's father had disappeared from his life when he was

3 years old, and his mother was left to take care of him and two older brothers. She worked two jobs, and in between she was always out at the bars looking for men. He grew up feeling that his mother really didn't care about him. If she did, she would not have kept leaving him with his uncle for the weekend even after he told her he didn't like him. Jake concluded very early in his life that "I'm not worth caring about."

Suicidality

According to the National Center for Victims of Crime, one-third of female survivors of rape have seriously contemplated suicide—four times more than non–crime victims. And female rape victims are 13 times more likely to attempt suicide than nonvictims. Survivors of childhood sexual abuse and assault are at even greater risk for suicidal thoughts and attempts.

Guilt and Shame

Guilt and shame are frequent emotional reactions to sexual assault and abuse. Guilt is about feeling responsibility for personal actions. Survivors frequently focus on what they could have done to prevent or escape from the assault—this naturally gives them a greater sense of control and makes the whole thing seem less frightening. Tess felt responsible for the sexual assault because she had worn a short skirt and makeup, drunk alcohol, and flirted with Campbell. She also thought that it never would have happened if she hadn't gone to the back room. She was just trying to "loosen up" and have a good time, but one thing led to another, and the next thing she knew she was trapped and couldn't get away from them. She probably should have stuck close to Ariel, since Ariel knew what to expect at the frat parties. She thought it was all her fault for wanting to have a good time and hoping to meet a guy. Trying to understand how the assault happened helped her feel she could prevent another assault from happening in the future. This helped her feel that she had control over bad things happening, but it also may have contributed to her developing PTSD. When she blamed herself for what happened, Tess felt bad about herself. Consequently she avoided thinking about the rape whenever possible. As a result, she didn't have much opportunity to process things further and resolve the fear underlying her nightmares and intrusive memories.

Jake remembered that the first time his uncle touched him he had invited him to play a game. Jake had thought the game was fun, so he wanted to keep playing. And at first he liked spending time with his uncle—ever since his father left, he had had no real attention from a man, and his mother wasn't really much fun to be with. So at first he thought it felt good to get all the attention. When his uncle sat him on his lap and started to touch him, he knew it didn't feel right, but he went along with it anyway. Jake was sure it was all his fault—if he had just told him no, then none of it would have happened.

Shame can range from mild embarrassment to a painful and debilitating sense of having lost personal integrity, moral virtue, and self-esteem. Tess always had been a "good girl." She studied hard in school and didn't go out much—she didn't really have an interest in drinking and hadn't had much time for dating. In fact, she realized she was a bit behind her peers socially because she had been a virgin before the night at the frat house party. She hadn't been too concerned, though, because she knew that school was the most important thing, and she figured that eventually she would meet a guy who was right for her. Since the rape, though, she didn't want to be seen at all. She was so ashamed of what had happened that she couldn't look anyone in the eye. She thought everyone at school knew what had happened and thought she was a slut. She wasn't exactly saving herself for marriage, but she wanted her first sexual experience to be with someone who cared about her. She realized she had made a big mistake going into the back room with Tommy. And, although she had been interested in Campbell, she was mortified that he had made her perform oral sex on him. She had barely ever kissed a guy, let alone done *that*—she thought that was something only prostitutes did, and she saw it as disgusting. How could she ever look either of them in the eye again? She sat in the back of the room in chemistry class to prevent Tommy and his friends from looking at her. She thought he had been her friend, but now every time she saw him in class she relived the whole thing and felt dirty. Who has sex with three guys all at once? It was utterly disgraceful! She felt damaged. What nice guy would ever want to date her now?

Even though they weren't at school with her, Tess's parents, Maggie and Ian, knew the assault was hard on her. They noticed a difference in how she talked with them on the phone, and when she came home on the weekends it was clear that she was depressed and felt bad about herself. They tried to be supportive, but she really didn't explain much about what had happened, so what could they do? Their once vibrant and fun daughter had become a social recluse.

Jake's shame went right to the core of who he was. Ever since he could remember, he had thought of himself as "dirty" and "bad" and "worthless." He thought his uncle had molested him because he could see what a perverted kid he was. And his mother not protecting him? Well, that just showed him how really worthless he was. The way he saw it, even his own mother didn't think he was worth protecting. As he got older, he started to do bad things at school—what did it matter anyway? Everyone knew what a good-for-nothing he was. Over time, his shame and the negative thoughts about himself because of the sexual abuse became a sort of self-fulfilling prophecy. Jake never believed that he deserved anything good or was worthy enough to be around decent people. So he spent most of his time with friends who engaged in dangerous, illegal behavior, and when bad things happened to him as a result it was just more proof that he didn't deserve anything good.

Substance Abuse

Women who survive sexual assault are much more likely to abuse alcohol and illicit drugs than those who have not been victimized. Typically, they use drugs to manage symptoms related to the assault. Marcy, who had been raped at a bar downtown, had tried many medications in an effort to decrease her anxiety, but marijuana was all that seemed to help. She knew it was illegal, but it was the only thing that worked, so she didn't feel like she had a choice. You may have noticed that your loved one drinks or uses drugs more since the sexual assault. She may drink more when she has to go into public places or be around people, in an effort to calm herself so that she can get through the situation. Estelle used alcohol to try to keep her mind off the sexual assault, and to help herself sleep. Unfortunately, alcohol and drug use is one factor that leads sexual abuse and assault survivors to further victimization.

Dissociation

A person who mentally disconnects from the real world is said to be "dissociating." The disconnection with reality can range from a mild sense of things being unreal or feeling "spacey" to being mentally in a different time or place than where one physically is. In the extreme, a person may have no recollection of where she was during the period of dissociation. Dissociation is one of the most confusing aspects of trauma for loved ones to understand. Often you can recognize that a person is dissociating because her eyes will appear glazed over and she may be minimally or completely unresponsive to your attempts to communicate with her. Some dissociative episodes might involve a "flashback" in which the person is reexperiencing the trauma to such an extent that she loses connection with the reality of the present. She may speak or act in ways that she did during the traumatic event, as if she is transported back in time to that moment. At other times, dissociation may simply involve disconnecting from the here and now, with no signs that the person is feeling distressed. You can think of dissociation as being an extreme form of daydreaming. You might have had a time when you had a lot on your mind that you were thinking about while driving somewhere. When you arrived at your destination, you realized that you didn't notice anything along the way. This can happen because our brains are capable of functioning on "automatic pilot." We can carry out routine tasks without careful thought while our mental focus is on other things.

Scientific understanding of dissociation is still in its infancy. Anybody can engage in dissociation, especially people with vivid imaginations. It may come as no surprise to you that teenagers are particularly prone to daydreaming and dissociative behaviors. Scientists believe, however, that intensely frightening and overwhelming aspects of traumatic experiences can elicit dissociative reactions in some people. Dissociating during a traumatic event (called *peritraumatic dissociation*) is among the strongest predictors of later developing PTSD.

Dissociation during the event can range from feeling spacey, unreal, unfamiliar, or disconnected to feeling outside of one's body, watching the event like another person, going somewhere else in one's mind, or completely "disappearing." In rare instances, the survivor may have had little or no memory of the event. As a result, she may not have been bothered by memories or felt a need to avoid reminders since the event happened. Larissa had dissociated when her cousin was molesting her, which had interfered with her ability to recall the abuse even though it always had affected her life. Jessie, who had been molested by her grandfather, learned to retreat to a "fantasy land" in her mind where she hid while the abuse was happening. She was powerless at the time, so mental escape was her only option. Later in her life she found that her memories of the abuse were fragmented and disorganized.

Intense dissociation may be related to the extent of uncontrollability the survivor experienced during the event, and it appears to be more common among children suffering something traumatic. Childhood sexual abuse frequently involves feeling trapped, restrained, and powerless and can be very frightening, so it makes sense that a child learns to resort to this very simple method of mentally surviving the event. Dissociation may become a habit for some victims who experience repeated episodes of trauma. They may be strongly triggered to dissociate when faced with reminders of the trauma in daily life, which can be a daily occurrence for some trauma survivors. In severe cases, the trauma survivor may "lose" blocks of time on a regular basis, which can be frightening and disturbing to both the survivor and her loved ones.

Sexual Functioning

Sexual assaults and abuse can have profound effects on the sexual functioning and intimacy of survivors. These effects can vary widely. Some survivors are anxious and fearful about physical intimacy and avoid it in ways that range from discomfort with certain intimate behaviors, sexual acts, or sexual positions to complete avoidance of all physical contact. They may avoid being touched in a certain way to avoid memories of the assault. The man who raped Marcy in the bar had kissed her neck repeatedly, and she was revolted by his smell and the feeling of his beard on her neck. Marcy continued to date men after this happened, but whenever her partner kissed her neck she went out of her way to change positions so he couldn't do that. She never dated men with beards, and if a guy she was dating started to grow one she would cajole him into shaving it off. If the guy she was seeing seemed to really like kissing her neck, she usually just ended up dropping him even if she really liked him—she just couldn't tolerate being reminded in that way.

Some survivors experience complete absence of libido—a total loss of interest in sex—while others are simply unable to relax enough to enjoy sexual relations. Ever since she was attacked, Estelle didn't seem like herself anymore. She used to be easy to be with, loving, and fun. She and Juan had always had made a point of having a "date night" at least once a week. He went out of his way to be romantic, and she had always enjoyed being intimate. After the assault, she refused to go out for a night on the town with him. And when they stayed home to cuddle in front of the TV, she no longer seemed comfortable sitting close to him. Usually she drank a few beers and passed out. Their sex life had been practically nonexistent since the assault. Juan was sad about what they had lost and frustrated at not being able to get the old Estelle back.

Men may have difficulty achieving an erection, and women may be unable to have an orgasm. After his father died when he was 11 years old, Omar's mother made him sleep in bed with her. As he got older, she started touching him in bed, which made him uncomfortable. The only way he could have any control was to learn to suppress his erection. Now, as an adult, he found he was unable to have an erection with his wife. She seemed okay with this and wasn't very interested in sex herself, but he was extremely frustrated and dissatisfied with their lack of a sex life. As a result of being molested by her babysitter, Pamela felt frozen inside when it came to being close with her boyfriends. She enjoyed dating and getting to know them, but as soon as they tried to get closer she felt numb. She knew they could tell, and they usually lost interest in her. Even when she tried to go further to satisfy her partner, she couldn't really respond to his touch, and she had never had an orgasm, even though she was 35 years old. Most of the time, her relationships had just slowly dissolved, and she suspected it was because her boyfriends didn't find her much fun in the bedroom. This made her sad and, until she met her fiancé, Caleb, she was afraid that she would be alone her whole life. Caleb was her first partner who really seemed to appreciate her as a whole person and didn't seem put off by the difficulties she had. This motivated her to work really hard in therapy to change old habits and resolve her sexual problems.

In some cases the survivor may engage in promiscuous or unsafe sex or experience confusion about his sexual orientation. In her 20s, before she met Carlos, Larissa had drunk a lot and gone out to bars several nights a week, often taking a different guy home with her each time. She liked having their attention. She was so drunk she hardly noticed the sex anyway, and if she did she just numbed out until it was over. The best part was that she felt wanted, because the rest of the time she didn't feel very attractive or connected to anyone. Things changed after she met Carlos—for the first time she felt like a guy really enjoyed her company. So she made an effort to cut back on her drinking and be a good partner to him, but she could never quite be mentally present when they had sex. She thought she had done a pretty good job of being a good wife, though, in spite of the effort it took just to let him touch her.

Other Negative Results

Sometimes sexual assault or abuse can have other unwanted effects for the survivor. These can include pregnancy or a sexually transmitted disease (STD) as a result of the assault or suffering serious injuries that leave scars, marks, or impairment in functioning. Pregnancy can result in ethical and emotional conflicts for the survivor and can be particularly difficult when the survivor is a minor and when the perpetrator is a family member. If your loved one is faced with decisions about an unwanted pregnancy resulting from an assault, your nonjudgmental compassion and support of her decisions are critical. These are situations where professional guidance is invaluable in helping to resolve the conflicts.

Your loved one may be dealing with the aftereffects of an untreated STD, which may have repercussions for her life. Sexually transmitted diseases warrant medical attention—if left untreated they can have long-term health consequences, including infertility, cancer, chronic illness, and even death. Once again, your support and understanding are critical, and seeking professional help in coping with these effects can be beneficial. Finally, your loved one might have suffered marks, scars, or impairments in function as a result of the assault, and these can magnify problems coping with the aftermath. After a sexual assault that included anal penetration, Sinead experienced intense discomfort and bleeding when she used the bathroom, and her physician informed her that she was bleeding from two deep lacerations inside her. She was horrified by the injuries that she had sustained and felt tremendous anger at her assailant not only for taking her power away and violating her but also for damaging her body.

Are There Problems Specific to Childhood Sexual Abuse?

As with sexual assault, all of the problems we described in Chapter 2 that can be caused by trauma can be caused by sexual abuse. Unfortunately, sexual abuse often is associated with a wide range of problems for those who survive it.

General Effects of Childhood Sexual Abuse

Estimates are that 20–30% of women and perhaps as many as 15% of men experienced some form of sexual abuse in childhood. Sexual abuse experiences, and the survivor's reactions to them, can vary widely. Whereas some survivors of sexual abuse experience minimal or even inconsequential distress, others experience severe problems and difficulties functioning in many areas of life. As with other forms of trauma, resilience is the norm—as many as 20–40% of adult survivors of childhood sexual abuse report no residual effects. About 20–30% of survivors of sexual abuse will experience significant and lasting negative effects similar to the problems of adult sexual assault survivors. These can include the reexperiencing and hyperarousal associated with PTSD, general anxiety and fears, and problems with low self-esteem, shame, and depression. Some of the problems discussed above—dissociation, substance abuse, and increased risk for suicide—are actually more common among survivors of childhood sexual abuse than among those who experience sexual trauma only in adulthood.

Other Effects of Childhood Sexual Abuse

In addition to the general effects of trauma, survivors of childhood sexual abuse experience some problems that are specific to sexual abuse or more likely to affect those who survive it. Child sexual abuse survivors often show **earlier physical maturation**, with earlier onset of menstruation, precocious sexual behaviors, exhibitionism, and attempts to seek sexual contact from older children or adults. Earlier sexualization often leads to promiscuity among sexually abused girls and increases risk for teen pregnancy. Both male and female child sexual abuse survivors engage in **more risk-taking behaviors** and have been found to be at increased risk for future sexual assaults. The tendency to isolate can lead to significant **problems in interpersonal relationships**. This is not unique among trauma survivors, but child sexual abuse survivors often isolate out of profound **mistrust of others** and severe **social anxiety**, which can be related to shame and negative perceptions of themselves as a whole person.

Eventually, as Jake got older, he spent less time with "troublemakers" and settled into a job in a supermarket, where he worked his way up to manager of the produce department. He met Lisa at work, and she was attracted to him from the start—she liked his sensitive, caring nature and didn't mind that he was "quiet." On the outside, life seemed normal for a while. It wasn't until they had been married for 8 years and their son, Cody, was almost school age that Lisa started to notice changes in Jake. He had always been "moody," but lately he was downright snappy. He seemed to avoid spending time with Cody and never wanted to go out with their friends anymore. His drinking was starting to seem out of control. Plus, he didn't seem to care about being intimate anymore—she couldn't even remember the last time they had had sex. Their relationship was in trouble until she insisted he go for therapy. Finally, a month into his therapy, he told her what was behind all these changes—that he had been molested as a kid and their son, having reached the age he was when the abuse started, was a constant reminder, dredging up all his old feelings that he thought he had tucked away.

Childhood sexual abuse survivors may be more likely than survivors of other types of trauma to experience the **problems with overall regulation of emotions** that we talked about in Chapters 2 and 3. They may feel as if they are on an emotional roller coaster with their moods swinging from one extreme to another many times in the course of a day. Jessie used dissociation to escape the horrifying experience of sexual abuse by her grandfather. Soon she developed a habit of employing dissociation to deal with other upsetting situations. As a result, she never really learned how to listen to and understand her own emotions. They always seemed out of her control, mostly because she hadn't developed any ways to soothe herself when she was distressed. Unable to understand or modulate her emotions, Jessie found that her feelings could range widely in a single day, and the people around her started to avoid her if she showed any kind of emotion.

Abuse by Fathers

Sexual abuse perpetrated by a father or stepfather tends to be more traumatic than abuse perpetrated by other family members. This may be because abuse by a parent usually occurs in the context of greater overall family dysfunction than abuse by others. As a result, less support may be available to the child, and it's more likely that the child will not be believed when she discloses the abuse to others. Also, when a parent is the abuser, there is a greater sense of betrayal and loss of trust. Finally, there may be greater family conflict and dissolution of family relationships when the father is the perpetrator of sexual abuse.

What Determines How a Survivor of Sexual Abuse Is Affected?

In general, more severe abuse is related to worse outcomes. For example, the longer the duration of the abuse, the more extreme the sexual acts involved, and the closer the relationship between the survivor and the perpetrator, the worse the effects of the sexual abuse will be. The survivor's response to the abuse and how she copes with it over the long term also are related to its effects. As we mentioned earlier, avoidance and dissociation during the abuse is related to greater risk of PTSD and distress in the long term. Overall, studies across many different groups of sexual abuse survivors consistently show that use of avoidant coping strategies, such as wishful thinking, self-criticism, and social withdrawal, is related to greater long-term distress. Jake thought the abuse by his uncle happened because of something about him, and he tended to criticize himself a lot. As noted earlier, this kept him locked in a pattern of harmful behavior and relationships and prevented him from having positive experiences and finding out that he really was a good person. The more severe the abuse is, the more likely the survivor is to use avoidant coping. Also, survivors who assume responsibility for the abuse and blame themselves for it are more likely to use avoidant coping strategies. This can happen, for example, when the abuse occurs repeatedly over long periods of time or at older ages. Self-blame also can happen in abuse situations where there is *less* use of force. When Pamela thought back to having been abused by a babysitter when she was 10, she could not remember trying to resist or fight. She basically went along with it, and she tended to take responsibility for this, as if she had caused or encouraged the sitter to molest her. When survivors perceive a high degree of stigma around sexual abuse, they also are more likely to use avoidant coping.

The ways that adults cope with their memories of childhood sexual abuse experiences also are strongly related to their well-being. Continued rumination about the abuse, including efforts to seek meaning, is a sign that the trauma is unresolved. Unresolved abuse is associated with avoidant coping strategies, which are related to feeling depressed. After her cousin died, Larissa no longer was afraid of him, but she also felt like she had no way to get "closure" on the abuse from her childhood. She found herself actually feeling sad that he had died because it meant that she had lost the opportunity to confront him about what he did. She thought that if only she could have gotten some sort of explanation from him, she would somehow be less bothered by what he had done. Instead, she thought about the abuse a lot and felt unfulfilled. In contrast, adults who have found meaning in their experiences are less distressed and less socially isolated. They tend to have higher self-esteem and better overall adjustment than those who are still seeking meaning. You may recall from Chapter 3 that Tess was able to recover from the rape and go on to support campaigns for better laws protecting women. She never felt glad that she had been raped, but she was able to grow from the experience and find something meaningful in her life as a result of it (we talk more about this in Chapter 12). If your loved one continues efforts to seek meaning related to the sexual assault or abuse, this is a clue that there may be "unfinished business" that might be resolved in therapy.

Seeking social support, on the other hand, has been related to greater self-esteem and long-term well-being. The response of the support system, however, is the key to this relationship. As with adults, negative responses to disclosure of child abuse often affect the survivor negatively. When disclosure of sexual abuse is met with suspicion or doubt, the effect can be devastating to young children's sense of trust, especially if someone close to them, such as a parent, refuses to believe what they are saying. When a parent reacts to the disclosure by becoming involved in the child's healing process, the effects of the abuse tend to be less severe. As adults, survivors of childhood sexual abuse also may feel abandoned or judged if they are not supported when they disclose their experiences. Reactions of acceptance and kindness to disclosures of sexual abuse can mitigate the sense of isolation many abuse survivors feel. When Jessie told her boyfriend, Alex, that she had been molested by her grandfather and only now was remembering the main details, he was unsure how to react. He was honest about this with Jessie. "I'm not sure what to say or do," he said, "but I really care about you, so I'll try to help you in whatever way you want." Alex said it helped to realize that something was behind her moodiness. Jessie felt immense relief, and Alex, who still really wasn't sure how the abuse was affecting her, nonetheless felt like he had eased her pain a little bit. They felt closer to each other after the exchange.

Does Sexual Assault and Abuse Affect Men Differently?

Overall, women experience sexual assaults and abuse more often at all times of life than men do. This may be one reason women have higher rates of PTSD than men. Yet men do experience sexual assault and abuse, and when they do they can be affected as profoundly as women, though perhaps in slightly different ways. Most experts agree that sexual assaults among men are severely underreported. Research estimates that around 7% of men in the United States have been sexually assaulted in adulthood (see review by Tewksbury, 2007). Rates are two to three times higher for college students and even higher among homosexual men. As a result, some researchers have theorized the sexual assaults against men are accounted for primarily by the experiences of homosexual and bisexual men, in the form of assaults by acquaintances or former dating partners. This does not negate the fact, however, that heterosexual men also are victims of sexual assault, and sexual assaults against men are sometimes perpetrated by heterosexual men, as well as by women. Also, rates of childhood sexual abuse are high—around 12% of men have experienced some form of sexual assault or abuse at some point in their lives, and most experienced sexual abuse before age 18. As many as 65% of men who experienced a sexual assault as an adult also had been sexually abused as children. Not all sexual assaults of men involve anal penetration. But rapes against men are more likely to be violent and involve physical force and use of a weapon than those perpetrated against women, although women are more likely to be injured.

The sense of stigma, shame, and embarrassment associated with sexual assault is particularly heightened for men. As a result, men often cope in stoic ways and are unlikely to display emotional reactions to the assault. When they do, men are more likely than women to respond with hostility, not only toward the perpetrator but also toward those around them, even family and friends. Men, even more than women, anticipate that authorities would not believe them if they reported the assault, and they worry that their sexuality will be questioned. Shame often is related to self-blame for the assault. The combination of stigma, shame, and fear of rejection inhibits most men from reporting assaults to authorities or seeking medical or mental health assistance. Male survivors of sexual assault are at higher risk than other men for developing problems including anxiety, depression, alcohol and drug abuse, and violent behavior, and the likelihood of developing such problems is even higher for those victimized in childhood. Sexually assaulted men are more likely than female survivors to engage in self-harm behaviors, and this is particularly so for those sexually abused in childhood.

Male sexual assault survivors are more likely to suffer from severe depression and hostility than female survivors. Sexual assaults lead men to question their masculinity, sexuality, and overall sense of control in the world. They experience problems with low self-esteem, negative body image, sleep disturbance, fear of revictimization, heightened general anxiety, and suicidal thoughts and attempts, particularly among adolescent and young adult male sexual assault survivors. As with women, social withdrawal is common.

Sexual Assault in the Military

With more women entering the military, many women experience sexual assault as part of their military experience. Men also experience sexual assault in the military, at rates similar to those in the civilian world. The hierarchies of power, emphasis on violence, and restrictive aspects of military life may contribute to assaults in the military. Recent studies show that, compared to assaults before or after military service, sexual assaults that take place during military service have more severe effects. This might be because service members feel more trapped, because the sexual assault takes place in an environment with many other threats to safety, or because of the increased sense of betrayal that survivors of military sexual assault typically feel. Sexual harassment also is a problem experienced by many women and some men in military settings. This subject is covered in more depth in Chapter 10.

Sexual Assault and the Legal System

As we've noted, sexual assault is among the most severe types of traumatic experiences. Following the assault, the survivor often turns to medical and legal systems for help and support. And yet in many instances the survivor's experience with the legal system exacerbates her sense of powerlessness, shame, and guilt and can be considered an additional trauma (see Campbell, 2008). As we've discussed, others' reactions to disclosure can either be a buffer against mental health problems or a contributing factor, exacerbating shame and difficulties with trust and inhibiting processing of trauma memories. This also applies to reactions of personnel within the legal system. A supportive experience that results in a successful conviction and sentencing of the perpetrator can build a sense of control and empowerment for the victim. Unfortunately, only a small minority of sexual assault cases end with a legal conviction. The vast majority of cases never go to trial—most are weeded out in earlier stages of the legal process. Nonetheless, the survivors are subjected to a grueling and often dehumanizing process of interrogation that frequently puts them at greater risk for long-term emotional problems. During this process, sexual assault survivors often feel intimidated, blamed, and threatened. Even when their cases go to trial, they often find the experience frustrating, embarrassing, and distressing. Their contact with the legal system leaves them feeling bad about themselves, depressed, violated, mistrustful, and reluctant to seek help again.

Most sexual assaults are perpetrated by someone close to the victim, but cases in which the victim knew the assailant are much less likely to be prosecuted. Along the way, the assault survivor is questioned repeatedly, not only about the details of the assault but also about her own behavior and her sexual experiences prior to the assault, despite the fact that such information cannot be brought up in court. The experience of reporting the assault to the police and then having the case not move forward is associated with greater risk for PTSD. The assistance of a victim advocate from a rape crisis center can mitigate some of the harm done by contact with the legal system. As Tess worked through the rape with a therapist at her school's counseling center, she found out that the college had a rape crisis and support center, staffed by peer counselors. It took a lot of courage for her to go in and seek help, but she was accepted immediately by the women who worked there, and several of them disclosed that they too had been assaulted in the past. They offered to help Tess press charges if she wanted to, and she decided that regardless of the outcome she wanted to bring charges against the men who had raped her. The rape crisis center staff made sure she was never alone when she talked to the police and went to court. Unfortunately, the defense attorneys found witnesses who had seen Tess drinking a lot that night, and no one at the party could remember hearing her scream for help. The three men were not convicted, but in the end Tess felt like she had done the right thing, and the rape crisis center had helped her through the process step by step, which made the legal process less stressful for her.

The Importance of Support and Validation

As discussed above, research has shown that the survivor's emotional reactions and risk for mental health problems are strongly associated with how others respond to the disclosure of sexual assault or abuse. This is particularly true for female survivors. Lack of social support is more strongly related to the development of posttraumatic stress symptoms in women than in men. This suggests that social support may be particularly beneficial for female survivors of sexual assaults, abuse, or harassment. Support can come from community resources such as rape crisis centers or support groups, family members, friends, or the legal system.

Healing Is Possible

Survivors of sexual assault and abuse face many challenges as they move forward in their lives. We hope you've developed a better understanding of some of the issues with which your loved one may be struggling. As you've seen, the stigma associated with sexual assault leads many survivors down a path of increasing *disconnection* from others, whereas *connection* promotes healing. It is not your job to resolve these issues, but by understanding how they come about, you may be able to cultivate a compassionate and validating stance toward your loved one's struggles.

Do you remember the warning at the beginning of this chapter? If reading the explicit descriptions of sexual assault or sexual abuse was disturbing to you, think how it must feel for the survivors of these experiences. Your loved one might be struggling with such discomfort. The more you work through your own reactions to and judgments about sexual trauma and those who survive it, the better able you will be to relate to and support your loved one.

Many of the effects of sexual assault and abuse are best dealt with by a professional therapist. A skilled therapist will involve the survivor's partner, or in some cases will refer the couple to a couple's therapist to address issues that affect the relationship. The good news is that research has shown that treatment for PTSD can be very effective with survivors of sexual assaults *and* sexual abuse. Indeed, several of the treatments described in Chapter 4 have been studied extensively with survivors of sexual assault, and research tells us that they work. Even so, as you've seen, PTSD may not be the only problem the sexual abuse survivor is facing, but there are also effective treatments for many of the other problems, and more is known about what causes and perpetuates them than ever before. Armed with your increased awareness of how your loved one's problems might be connected to his assault and abuse experiences, you can help him move forward on a path toward healing.

TEN

When Someone You Love Has Been to War

What confused Jenny most about Marcus's behavior since he'd been back from Iraq was that he didn't seem proud of his military service anymore. The edginess in public places, the nightmares, the dislike of anyone who looked Muslim or Middle Eastern—that all made sense to Jenny, given what Marcus had experienced overseas. But he never put on his uniform anymore, and in fact he kept all his gear in a box in the attic where it was out of sight. When the war or the military came up in conversation, he didn't say anything. It seemed like he didn't even want to be reminded of the military. She couldn't understand—the military used to be such a big part of his life and of who he was. Now it seemed like he just wanted to be rid of it.

Zach had never understood the phrase "loose cannon" until his brother Hank got out of the Army. Hank had signed up for 4 years of service, but he was home after only 2½ years. Zach couldn't understand how that came about. Hank didn't seem to sleep much, and when he was awake he was starting an argument, getting drunk, sitting in front of his computer, or involved in some combination of those activities. He came off as angry at everyone and not caring about anything, but Zach knew his brother really well (they were only a year apart), and it seemed to him that Hank was scared and sad, and all that anger and recklessness was just Hank trying to pretend that he didn't care. Zach couldn't understand any of it. After all, Hank hadn't left American soil. What could have happened to him?

Eva had read that soldiers came back angry, but it felt like she was angrier than her husband. When Mark had gotten notice that he was being activated by the Guard and deploying to Afghanistan, she almost had to force him to sit down and discuss it with the kids. It had taken the boys a couple of months to adjust, but she had kept everything running smoothly, so they eventually settled into the new routine. It had been hard to run the household, go to work, and keep the reins on three boys, but, although it tired her out, she did it. She just kept reminding herself that it would be only a year and then Mark would be back. But when he came back, things didn't get better—in fact, they seemed to get worse. Not only was Mark of no help to her, his presence was like having another child in the home. He did nothing around the house and spent most of his days playing video games. Even worse, he was horribly lax with the boys—all he ever seemed to say was "Aw, they're young, don't worry about it!" He seemed to think that because he had served his country he should be waited on hand and foot. Eva was really pissed at him, and deep down, she knew that the one thing she had learned while he was gone was that he wasn't necessary— she could handle everything on her own. She found herself wondering whether she would be better off without him.

Kwame didn't have any idea how he should act around Gina anymore. He had thought that after 3 years together they could survive her deployment, but he was really struggling. Her moods were at the extremes—she was either really sad or really angry, sometimes both at the same time. She had punched people twice in bars, for reasons Kwame still couldn't understand, and fortunately she hadn't gotten into trouble either time. She always wanted him to be around but never wanted to be touched or have sex. He hated to think that her deployment could wreck all that they had, but he couldn't see the relationship going on like this. Something had to change.

Military trauma is unique in that the survivor experiences it in the context of serving in the armed forces. The effects of trauma that we discussed in Chapter 2 can be complicated by some of the specific features of military life. The world of soldiers, sailors, airmen, and Marines is so different from that of civilians that being in the military really is like living in a different culture. Service members who leave the military world and its culture typically must readjust to the civilian world, whether or not they were deployed to a war zone, experienced trauma, or even left the country. **For returning service members who have suffered trauma, the readjustment process multiplies the challenges that they and their loved ones face after deployment.** In this chapter we look at how readjustment struggles can compound symptoms of posttraumatic stress. Knowing whether your loved one's difficulties are related to readjustment or trauma can help you figure out what kind of help he needs. We also discuss the kinds of professional help available through veterans', military, and private sources for military personnel experiencing posttraumatic stress.

The Uniqueness of Military Culture

If you've spent a lot of time around military personnel, lived on a military base, or served in the military yourself, you've undoubtedly noticed some of the differences between military and civilian life. The armed forces have their own language, specific values, and rules for interpersonal relationships. Military bases are like self-contained countries, with their own laws, rules, grocery stores, and even movie theaters and bowling alleys.

In fact, if you haven't been exposed to the military, it might be easier to understand how different the military world is if you think of a soldier returning from service as somewhat like a person returning from an extended stay abroad. The purpose of such an experience, especially when it's part of an education, is to learn about a different way of life, so you would expect a returning civilian to develop new tastes in food, new ways of dressing, or a different perspective on his home country. Likewise, a soldier living on a military base, in his own country or abroad, typically is transformed by the experience. Returning service members have learned different customs, languages, and ways of looking at the world, just like returning travelers. Yet we often expect service members to be exactly as they were before they left. This expectation can set up the soldier for frustration and you for disappointment. Unlike civilian trauma survivors, service members and veterans recover from traumatic experiences in the context of postdeployment readjustment and/or return to civilian culture. This complicates our efforts to understand their struggle with posttraumatic stress.

The Critical Importance of Trust

One of the important differences between civilian and military cultures is the extent to which soldiers rely on and trust one another in the course of their work. The ultimate objective of a military unit is to function effectively as a team to survive the life-or-death situations inherent in war. Members of the armed forces undergo the intense trials of basic training together, and the military instills in soldiers a willingness and commitment to do anything for their fellow service men and women. Soldiers trust completely that the men or women around them will protect them at all costs. Teamwork, sacrifice, and total commitment to the job at hand are the mainstays of military life. These qualities also are widely valued in civilian life. Yet the bonds of trust among military personnel are strong and hard to match in the civilian world. Friendships that were strong prior to military service can be strained upon return home, when a civilian friend may feel like an outsider.

Many civilian employers recognize that, due to qualities instilled by military training and service, former service members often make excellent employees. Military veterans often demonstrate a high level of dedication to work objectives. They are disciplined, skilled problem solvers, and they understand the importance of teamwork. Yet the same qualities that make military service members desirable employees sometimes can interfere with their ability to keep a job. Many soldiers are surprised and confused to discover that the level of trust among service members does not exist in the civilian world. This realization can make it hard to trust civilians.

Reed served in the Army for 6 years. He knew he could trust his fellow soldiers to protect him regardless of the circumstances. Likewise, he would sacrifice his life for any of them. After he retired from the military, he went through three civilian jobs in a year. Reed saw that people were out for themselves, and he felt like he couldn't trust anyone, which made him feel dissatisfied with his workplace. On two jobs, Reed's performance was poor because he didn't rely on his coworkers and instead tried to do everything on his own. On the third job, once he realized that he wouldn't be able to trust anyone around him, he simply walked out at lunch one day and didn't go back. His girlfriend, Leslie, couldn't understand why he was sometimes distant toward her yet still seemed close with his military buddies; she tried to figure out what she had done to lose his trust. For Reed, his difficulty trusting civilians added to his vigilance. It seemed like sources of threat were everywhere, and it was hard for him to let his guard down and allow anyone to get close.

Aaron, who spent 4 years in the Marine Corps, knew exactly what his fellow "grunts" knew. He trusted that if any Marine was not up to snuff, all the Marines around him would make sure he learned what he had to, because all of their lives might depend on that Marine being able to do his job. Like Reed, Aaron was continually frustrated at his first civilian job. As Aaron worked hard to learn his position and do the best job he could as part of the team, it seemed to him that everyone else was trying to figure out how to get by doing the minimum required of them. Aaron quickly lost his enthusiasm for his work and went home every day feeling unfulfilled and alone. He soon started to have unwanted memories of his time in Afghanistan, and trying to cope with these on top of his disenchantment with work placed a major strain on him.

As mentioned above, the bonds of trust between service members often are so strong that civilians may feel excluded. Military personnel who serve together develop powerful friendships as a result of sharing intense experiences during training and deployments to distant places. After a deployment to Panama, Kieran returned to his hometown and reconnected with friends he had known since kindergarten. At first his friends were glad to see him, but they soon drifted away after Kieran talked a lot about how close he had become with his fellow Marines. Not surprisingly, when he tried to explain why he could never be as close with anyone else, his friends of 20 years were hurt. How could he say that he felt closer to people he had known for only 4 years when he had known them for most of his life?

A Language of Their Own

Another aspect of military culture that can set service members and veterans apart from civilians is the strange language that service members and veterans seem to speak. The military uses many abbreviations and acronyms to communicate efficiently. Just as a person who spends time in another country may continue to use foreign words when he returns, the speech of service members and veterans often is infused with military jargon. This language can be bewildering to those who are not familiar with the technical concepts that these terms signify. Ike was confused when he overheard his daughter, Karen, on the phone with a friend from the National Guard. She referred to the time that another soldier had been "outside the wire" when a bomb detonated. The "EOD" had to be summoned to clear the area before they could all return to the "fob." Her voice sounded tense, and at one point she started to cry. Ike wanted to talk to her and soothe her, but he couldn't understand what she was talking about. He felt confused and helpless.

If your loved one uses words or phrases that you don't understand, it's okay to ask him what he means. Service members and veterans know that civilians don't understand the things they're familiar with, and they usually don't mind explaining. The day after he overheard her, Ike told Karen he was concerned because she had been crying on the phone. When he asked her what on earth she had been talking about, Karen laughed. She explained to her father that being "outside the wire" meant being off-base on a mission, "*EOD*" stood for "explosive ordnance disposal," and "*fob*" was a "forward operating base." She said she didn't want to talk about what had happened that day, and Ike told her that if she ever changed her mind, he'd be willing to listen. Karen thanked him. Ike felt like he had been able to provide her some support, and it helped that he had been able to find out what she had been talking about.

Military versus Civilian Daily Life

Many other aspects of military life beyond the effects of living in a different culture can affect readjustment to the civilian world. Veterans who have separated from the military often feel burdened by demands of civilian life that they did not have to worry about when they were in the military. When their civilian family members don't understand how difficult it is for returning soldiers just to slip back into their former routines, resentments can build. The differences between daily life in the military and civilian worlds cause readjustment problems for most service members as they transition back from a war zone or out of the military. Posttraumatic symptoms greatly compound the stress of readjustment—dealing with both can severely strain your loved one's coping resources.

Trouble Handling Mundane Responsibilities

In the military, much of daily life is taken care of for service members, especially while deployed. Soldiers on deployment have very few concerns other than fulfilling their duties and surviving. During his year in Iraq, Marcus never had to worry about how clean his clothes were or what he would wear. He didn't have to pay rent or cook. When he returned home, he simply wasn't used to dealing with daily chores. It didn't occur to him to do laundry, and it took several months (and a number of missed payments) for him to get back in the habit of paying bills. Marcus struggled to balance the family budget and he started to avoid his checkbook. Jenny didn't realize that her husband was ashamed that he couldn't handle his own bank account when he had excelled at operating multimillion-dollar equipment. After what she thought was a reasonable adjustment period, Jenny started to think Marcus was just taking advantage of her willingness to pick up the slack. But for a veteran who had ably executed his duties in a war zone under hazardous conditions, the struggle with civilian responsibilities can be frustrating and embarrassing.

Lack of Excitement

When a returning soldier is showing signs of posttraumatic stress, there may be nothing more perplexing to family and friends than watching the soldier pursue danger and risk at home. Yet whereas in some ways the civilian world can be more stressful than military life, it also can be far more boring. After deployments, some soldiers become involved in high-risk, "adrenaline junkie" hobbies like skydiving to try to recapture the excitement they felt during training and combat. Younger veterans may spend extensive time playing war-themed or other violent video games as a way to simulate their military experiences. Darren was part of a tank crew in Iraq, and his training involved moving at high speeds and firing very large weapons. His civilian job as a mechanic simply didn't excite him. His wife, Melanie, noticed that after his return he often drove very fast, weaving in and out of traffic, which he never used to do. When Melanie asked why he was driving like that, Darren said he was trying to get the same rush that he felt when he was in Iraq. Melanie didn't know how to react: was this the same man who cried out in fear in his sleep when a motorcycle roared down the street in the middle of the night?

The Upheaval of Deployment

Military personnel who are deployed to another country experience numerous challenges when they return home.

Changing Roles

When the service member departs for an extended period of time, family roles usually change. Often other family members have to fill the service member's roles within the family in addition to their own. Children also may be asked to take on more chores. Eva assumed most of Mark's responsibilities and ran the household herself while he was in Afghanistan, taking over bill paying, car maintenance, and yard work, and the boys picked up more chores to help out. When the warrior returns, he and the family often expect that things will go right back to normal, but this usually is not the case. Often the family has adopted daily routines that exclude the service member. When the service member returns from deployment, family roles must be redefined to integrate the returning soldier back into the family life. This process often can take as much time and cause as much upheaval as the soldier's departure did.

Before he left for Iraq, Paul had taken care of everything relating to the cars and the bills. While he was gone, his wife, Amanda, took over these duties in addition to keeping up the house. Amanda found that she liked balancing the family's budget every month. She felt more in control of their finances than when Paul had been in charge of them. When he got back, Amanda let him know that she really liked paying the bills and wanted to keep doing so. Paul was initially fine with this, until Amanda made it clear that she expected him to take over one of her jobs. After some heated negotiations, Paul and the boys (who had really pitched in while he was gone) took over the laundry.

Disrupted Plans and Interrupted Paths

Many service members and their families do not realize that a 1-year deployment does not mean only one year of their lives will be affected. Paul's unit was issued orders to deploy to Iraq from June through June of the next year. They also were scheduled for premobilization activities for the 6 weeks before they deployed, which meant that Paul was gone for more than 13 months. He missed two seasons of his oldest son's little league games. Paul had taught his son how to play, and baseball was their favorite shared activity, so Paul felt like he had missed out on a major chunk of his son's youth.

Gina, who had joined the National Guard to fund her college education, was in her second year of completing a 4-year biology degree, with plans to go to medical school. She got the orders for her April deployment in late January, after she had already begun classes at the university. As a result, she was faced with the choice of either withdrawing from her classes and being idle for 2 months or staying in them and taking incompletes. Her professors recommended that she withdraw and start over when she got back, which Gina reluctantly did. When she returned from her deployment the following April, Gina had to wait another 2 months until the summer term started to resume her studies, and the courses she needed for her major were not offered until the fall. So her 1-year deployment set her graduation timeline back 20 months.

When deployments interfere with progress toward a specific goal, soldiers may feel like they have "lost" time and others have passed them by. Gina found out she was deploying when she was 20 and a sophomore in college. When she got back, she was 22 and completing her sophomore year. She was suddenly noticeably older than her peers and felt out of place among them. Many of her friends had graduated and were out working. Gina often felt like she had fallen behind and should be working instead of still taking classes. Elvin got his orders to deploy to Kuwait when his wife, Marisol, was 3 months pregnant. She gave birth just a few months into his time in Kuwait, and he did not see his daughter until she was 6 months old. Elvin felt like her first months on earth had been taken away from him. Needless to say, these disruptions in the course of life can magnify the struggles that returning soldiers wage with any trauma they have suffered.

Readjustment after Military Trauma

Now that you know some of the ways in which military and civilian cultures differ, we hope it's easier for you to understand how your loved one may struggle to reintegrate into the civilian world and how this can complicate the effects of trauma. Like other trauma survivors, service members who have experienced traumatic events can suffer from the posttraumatic reactions described in Chapter 2. They may reexperience the trauma in daily life or dreams, be in a perpetual state of "high alert," work hard to avoid reminders of the trauma, and feel emotionally numb or disconnected from others. Due to unique aspects of military life, however, traumatic experiences can affect service members in particular ways that can make it even harder for your loved one to put his life back together. Knowing what you're observing will help guide you in how to help and cope.

Watchfulness and Safety Behaviors

As members of the armed forces, military personnel are trained to be watchful and to defend themselves and their fellow service members. They are familiar with weapons and in fact often feel unprotected without one. Watchfulness is particularly important for survival in war zones, so those who return from deployment may have been living for extended periods in a high state of alert. As a result, members of the military who have experienced trauma often show **more pronounced hypervigilance and protective behaviors** than civilians. Due to their familiarity with and access to weapons they may be more likely to incorporate them into their safety behaviors. Zach knew his brother Hank owned several handguns and a shotgun, but he was shocked when Hank told him that he rarely left the house without one of his firearms. When Zach asked why, Hank looked at him like he was crazy. "The world is dangerous, little brother," he said, "and I'm not gonna be the guy caught without a weapon." Similarly, one morning Kwame found a knife under Gina's pillow. She said that she always kept a knife there, "in case something happens." When Kwame asked what could happen, Gina seemed to get angry at him for not understanding.

Keep in mind that the service member or veteran in your life has been trained extensively in how to maintain, handle, and use a variety of weapons. His level of comfort with weapons is likely to be far higher than yours, but so will his respect for weapons and what they can do. If you are concerned about having weapons in the home, however, you have the right to express this to your loved one. The guidelines for assertive behavior described in Chapter 8 may help you reach a compromise about weapons.

Fear of Loss

Veterans and military personnel who have lost people close to them while deployed may be particularly **fearful of being close with others**. Before Marcus was deployed to Iraq, he had been very close with his daughter, Marion. Jenny noticed that Marcus was more distant from Marion after his return, and she couldn't understand why. Even though he loved Marion very much, Marcus was fearful of staying close to her, because, during his deployment, people he cared about were killed. If anything happened to her, he wasn't sure he would be able to handle it, so he kept her at a distance.

Mistrust of Authority

Military duty, by its nature, entails following orders. When things go wrong, service members often conclude that the orders they were given caused the negative events, and they may blame the person who gave the orders. As a result, they may believe that it is **unwise to trust people in authority**, which can lead to problems at work and in other situations in daily life. Gina knew that taking the same road every day for a week made her unit's movements predictable and therefore put them in danger. But her commanding officer continued to order them along the same route, and on the eighth day they were attacked. Gina blamed the officer for the attack. After she was discharged, she had a hard time following orders from bosses, which led to her losing several jobs. Related to their distrust of authority, some soldiers are suspicious of people who have only "book learning" and have not accumulated real-world experience. Gina thought her commanding officer made poor decisions because he didn't have enough field experience. As a result, she was suspicious of people in authority who came to their positions because of schooling and not on-the-job training. Her job performance suffered because she was reluctant to follow instructions of supervisors she didn't trust.

Disconnection from Civilians

Many soldiers believe that people who have never served in the military do not understand how the world *really* is. As a result, they may have **difficulty relating to civilians**. After she left the Army, Darci noticed that when she spent time with civilians she struggled to find things to talk about. She couldn't relate to their stories about office work and ball games, and she didn't think they understood her stories about the Army. A month after Marcus returned from Iraq, he overheard two men complaining about the soaring cost of gas. Marcus had lived in several other countries and knew that gas was still less expensive in America than it was in most other countries. He also had just returned from a place where civilians had no electricity or plumbing, had limited access to food, and lived in danger every day. He felt an urge to yell at the men to appreciate how lucky they were to live here.

Veterans who have been deployed to a war zone gain firsthand knowledge of how horrible war truly is. Civilians, by contrast, know war primarily through television, movies, and books, which tend to minimize the terrible aspects of war and focus on the more romantic and heroic elements. This glamorization of war can make veterans feel extremely uncomfortable around civilians who presume they know what it might have been like to be there but really have no idea. Todd had been part of an Army detachment responsible for clearing buildings using grenades before soldiers entered them. When they entered one building, Todd and his team found the remains of three children along with those of several insurgents and a large stash of weapons and maps. When a neighbor found out that Todd had been in Iraq, he asked him whether he was "kicking down doors and kicking asses." Todd wanted to tell him that he threw a grenade that blew up three young children, just to shut him up. But he realized that a civilian would not understand that he had made the correct decision by following established procedure even though it resulted in the deaths of three innocent children. He figured the guy would just label him a baby-killer because he wouldn't understand that soldiers often have to do horrible things in war. So Todd simply nodded and smiled and promised himself he would never speak to that neighbor again.

If you have never served in the military, then you most likely will *not* be able to understand all the things your loved one has experienced. Pretending that you do understand might only push your loved one further away. It can help to understand that the survivor's detachment from you is probably not personal; she probably reacts that way to most civilians. If you convey an honest interest in what she experienced during her military service, and if you allow her to decide how much she will disclose, you will open the door for her to feel more connected to you.

Anger

As we discussed in Chapter 2, trauma survivors often have difficulty managing anger, which can cause significant problems in their relationships. Among returning warriors and veterans, **anger can be even more intense.** Service members are trained to respond swiftly and decisively to threats, and anger often serves as a motivating force for this aggression. When confronted with a situation that he perceives as threatening, the survivor of military trauma is more likely to respond with aggression because that is what he has been trained to do. Zach noticed that Hank couldn't laugh things off, and he never showed fear. Instead, he reacted to most situations with intense anger, which would either intimidate the other person into a retreat or start a fight.

Discomfort with Public Reaction

People who have never served in the military sometimes ask questions that seem appropriate to them but that military personnel and veterans often find offensive or disrespectful. Once a neighbor asked Marcus why he wasn't still in Iraq fighting the war. Another time a man in a bar asked him what it was like to kill someone. These questions made Marcus so uncomfortable that he started avoiding talking to anyone outside of his close circle of family and friends. Many soldiers also can **feel uncomfortable at public ceremonies, parades, or memorials.** Mark had lost men close to him during his deployment, and he often wondered whether he could have done something to save them. When people thanked him for his service during the war, he thought about how he had failed to bring all his men back with him and felt like he didn't deserve to be thanked. As a result, he skipped events that honored veterans. This was puzzling to Eva, who was proud of his service and thought he should be too.

In the same way that it can help to let the service member or veteran in your life decide what he tells you about his military experiences, it also often is best to allow him to decide when he discloses his military service to others. Allow your loved one to control who knows that he served and how much they know about his service. This will allow him to develop ways of handling these issues in his conversations with others.

Anxiety around Certain Groups of People

Service members who had been deployed to hostile areas can experience **anxiety around people who remind them of the war zone.** Roger, who served in Vietnam and hadn't received treatment for his posttraumatic symptoms, had great difficulty being around Asian Americans, especially those of Vietnamese descent. Marcus became extremely anxious around people with Middle Eastern features. Once he made his whole family move their seats in a crowded movie theater when a man wearing a turban sat behind them. Veterans usually are aware that most Americans are not dangerous, but in the moment, seeing people who remind them of enemy combatants can be very frightening.

Battle Injuries and Scars

War is by nature violent and dangerous, and many soldiers are injured in the line of duty. The resulting **physical scars and injuries are daily reminders of war experiences.** Darren lost two fingers of his left hand in a bomb blast. Part of him was glad that he was right-handed, and he was proud of how well he had adjusted. But still, he was affected by the loss in many ways. Suddenly, simple activities like tying his shoes, buttoning his shirt, or snapping a photograph had become challenges. Every time he had to compensate for his missing digits he found himself wishing, despite all the progress he'd made, that he had his fingers back. A piece of shrapnel left a scar on Maria's abdomen. This didn't impair her life at all. Yet each morning when she stepped out of the shower and saw it in the mirror, she felt a pang of grief as she was reminded of the two men killed in the same explosion. When her friends talked about how they avoided watching the news because it reminded them of their deployments, Maria shook her head in frustration. She was carrying around a reminder of the war everywhere she went.

Guilt

Soldiers who experienced combat can feel **guilt** in several different ways. First, a service member may feel **guilty about something he did**. During the initial fighting in Iraq, Darren was involved in intense combat in which he killed at least six men. He sometimes found himself wondering who those men were. Did they have families? Were they soldiers or citizens fighting for their land and country? Sometimes he thought that killing them was wrong, and when he did he felt guilty.

The pressures experienced by service members in the war zone can be immense. They often have to ignore their fear and enter situations they know to be dangerous. They may see friends injured and killed, and they often are limited by rules of engagement that their enemies do not heed. Service members in war zones sometimes feel like they have no control over their thoughts, emotions, or behavior. They may go for long periods feeling so little control over anything that, occasionally, when they do get a chance to exert power, they grossly exceed what is appropriate for the situation. When a soldier witnesses four friends shot by a sniper in a single week, his anger and frustration may build. When his unit finally catches the sniper, it can be very difficult for him to treat that prisoner with dignity and respect. Later, when reflecting on their behavior in the war zone, warriors who used excessive violence often feel ashamed of their behavior. They may not recall the amount of pressure they were under or the intense emotions they experienced that influenced what they did.

Soldiers also sometimes feel **guilty about *not* having done something** that might have prevented a bad event from happening. While on patrol one night, Reed noticed a woman and two children walking quickly and turning down a narrow alley. He was suspicious of what they might be doing after dark, but he didn't investigate, assuming that a woman with children would not be a threat. Minutes later, a large explosion rocked the building on the other side of the alley, killing several local civilians. No one had been seen in the area except the woman and children, and Reed realized that the woman, who must have brought the children along with her for cover, had to have set the bomb. He felt guilty because he didn't try to stop her, and he blamed himself for the deaths of the civilians.

Finally, service members can feel **guilty about having survived** when others did not, such as when Marcus walked away from an explosion without a scratch even though his buddy was killed. A soldier with survivor guilt struggles to understand why he is still alive yet another soldier, maybe someone with children or plans for the future, no longer lives. The soldier may conclude that he has to live a certain way or accomplish certain things to make his life "worth" the other soldier's death.

The film *Saving Private Ryan* tells a story of survivor guilt from World War II. In the story, a team of soldiers is sent to find Private James Ryan and bring him out of the war zone because three of his brothers have been killed in the war, leaving him as the only surviving son in his family. In the course of retrieving him, numerous soldiers, including Captain John Miller, are killed. The film tells the story as James Ryan recalls it many years later while visiting a military cemetery as an older man. When he arrives at Captain Miller's grave, Ryan expresses his guilt about the men who sacrificed their lives to bring him home, revealing the incredible burden he has felt to make use of the life that others died to give him. "I tried to live my life the best that I could," he confesses to the grave. "I hope that was enough. I hope that, at least in your eyes, I've earned what all of you have done for me."

Soldiers who are sent home from the war zone for any reason, such as severe injuries that prevent them from completing their duties, sometimes feel guilty about not staying to help their buddies who are still there. Initially, when Captain Miller and his men finally located Private Ryan and informed him of their mission, he refused to go with them because he did not want to leave the men in his unit. Ryan didn't think it would be fair for him to go home if his colleagues could not. When Captain Miller asked him how they should explain to his mother that he refused to go home, Private Ryan replied, "You can tell her that when you found me, I was with the only brothers I had left. And that there was no way I was deserting them. I think she'd understand that." When Steve was sent home from Iraq after having been unconscious for 12 hours after a truck accident, he tried to keep track of his unit's location and progress from home. After a while, he had to stop. He didn't want to, because he felt like he was abandoning them.

But it was just too painful to get news about them when he was stuck at home, unable to help.

Besides feeling guilty about being unable to fight alongside his fellow Marines, Steve felt ashamed because his wounds weren't visible to others. It seemed to him that when others learned he had been sent home from Iraq due to injuries, the first thing they did was look him up and down, trying to see his wounds. His body was still in great shape—it was his brain that was the problem. Steve felt broken and defective. Many warriors are unable to serve in the war zone because of debilitating wounds that others can't see, such as PTSD and aftereffects of concussions sustained in accidents or explosions. Steve thought that Marines who came home on crutches or with arms in slings had legitimate reasons for being out of the war zone, but he felt like *he* was a fraud for not being over there.

You may be tempted to try to convince your loved one that he is not responsible for what happened. This is an understandable motivation, but be warned that it's very difficult to argue someone out of blaming himself for something, especially if you were not there. A couple of years after he got back, Reed confided in Leslie about the bombing that was the focus of his guilt. Leslie couldn't understand how he could blame himself for that. She told him that it wasn't his fault. After all, it was a war, and people set off bombs in wars. Wasn't it the bomber's fault? Reed just shook his head, got up, and left, and they didn't talk for the rest of the night. Leslie was mystified—why was he so insistent on blaming himself? She couldn't understand that Reed believed he should have been able to stop the bombing, and Leslie's words only reinforced this. It *was* a war—he should have been on the lookout. If a loved one opens up to you about guilt, it can be helpful to tell him that you understand how hard that must be and that you appreciate him trusting you enough to confide in you. Try not to judge what he is saying. Instead, recommend that he talk to someone who can help him work through his feelings.

Moral Confusion

Combat trauma often is complicated by the fact that the survivor intentionally killed other people. For soldiers who take life, intentionally or not, the problems caused by fear response to threatening situations are compounded by the complexities of adjusting to having killed others. The act of killing goes against beliefs about right and wrong taught by society and religion. Soldiers who kill not only sometimes feel guilty but also may question their beliefs about the world. When Mark came back from Afghanistan, he no longer went to church with his wife and kids. He couldn't sit in a place where he was constantly told that killing was wrong after he had killed to serve his country. For some soldiers, killing in the course of normal duty does not cause as much difficulty as killing in more complicated or ambiguous situations. Todd had few second thoughts about the seven insurgents he shot during firefights. They were clearly shooting at him, and he could tell himself quite truthfully that it was them or him. And heck, that was what was *supposed* to happen in war. But the deaths of the three children who were killed by the grenade he threw were *not* supposed to happen. When Todd decided to seek treatment, he had to work on the beliefs about what he did as well as the intrusive memories of various firefights.

As with guilt, you may find yourself tempted to tell your loved one that what she did was okay, that she had no choice, or that she was justified given the situation. Moral questions have to be worked out by the person asking them. You may find that taking a stance that counters your loved one's feelings about the situation accomplishes little, other than putting you in opposition to her. In responding to such moral conflicts, your best bet is to acknowledge both sides of the issue. Keith told Todd that he knew children do sometimes die in war and he understood how hard it was for Todd to accept his role in that. At the same time he emphasized how proud he was of him for having the courage to serve his country. When your loved one is struggling with moral confusion, it's wise to encourage her to talk this over with someone experienced in these issues whom she trusts, such as a counselor or a religious leader.

Loss of Identity

During transitions from the war zone back to a military base and the civilian world, service members often **struggle with losing their sense of identity**. After serving for many years in the military, and especially after long deployments to a war zone, it can be very hard to let go of the warrior identity. The dramatic differences between the military and civilian worlds can make it harder for the retiring soldier to bridge the two periods of her life. Some veterans resolve this by trying to stay as connected as possible to their military identities. After Darren left the Army, he spent time only with others who had served in the Army. He kept his truck covered with stickers from the countries where he had been deployed and the units with which he had served. Darren wore fatigues whenever he could and volunteered at a VA medical center in his spare time. He spent most evenings at the VFW, mingling with veterans from all eras.

Marcus, on the other hand, did not like the questions and recognition that always came when people found out he was a veteran. He also had conflicting feelings about some of the things he saw and did while deployed. So Marcus tried to distance himself from the military and all of his experiences with it. He kept his gear and awards in a cardboard box in the attic and didn't belong to any veterans' organizations. For Jenny, this was the reverse of how he had been before he had deployed—he had been proud of serving his country and never hesitated to tell other people about his involvement in the military. She couldn't see the distress that reminders of his time in Iraq caused him, so she couldn't understand why he was avoiding the military.

Mixed Emotions

Many service members and veterans leave their military experiences with a confusing mix of feelings. For many, the traumatic events they experienced in the military are the worst things that ever happened to them. Whether or not they suffer from PTSD, they may have experienced horrifying events that they would like to put behind them. What is confusing for these men and women, however, is that very often the military also is the source of the *best* experiences of their lives. Darren, who had been part of a tank crew, never felt as powerful as he did when he was in the military. Wayne had never left his hometown before he joined the Navy, and in 6 years he saw parts of the world that he had never heard of. While she was in the National Guard, Karen had made incredibly close friendships. Some of the best memories in her life were of things she had seen and accomplished with her fellow soldiers on different bases around the world. It can be hard to understand how something could have been so wonderful and so horrible at the same time. The good memories associated with the military can make avoidance doubly painful; by avoiding things that remind them of the military, many veterans also are avoiding some of their most treasured memories.

Noncombat Trauma

As we discussed earlier, perceptions of military experience can differ markedly from reality. When civilians think about military trauma, they usually picture combat scenarios similar to what they have seen on TV or in movies. Although it's true that combat-related events are the most frequent types of trauma experienced by members of the armed forces, service men and women also experience other types of potentially traumatic events. Soldiers on active duty often use heavy machinery, large vehicles, weapons, and explosives. As in any work-place, accidents sometimes occur during training exercises and normal duties, as well as in the war zone. When tools of war are involved, the consequences of such accidents can be horrific. In 2 years serving on the flight deck of a large aircraft carrier, Lance had seen two helicopters, each with several crew members, tumble off the side of a ship into the ocean. He also had witnessed jet exhaust set fire to a young recruit who stood too close to an aircraft as the pilot started the engines. Steve awoke in an Army hospital frustrated to realize that the injuries that landed him there were not incurred in an explosion or gunfire. Rather, the supply truck he was riding in had careened off the road into a ditch and flipped over while swerving to avoid other vehicles on a narrow road outside of Ramadi.

Men and women also sometimes experience sexual assault while serving in the military. A sexual assault by another member of the armed forces can be profoundly damaging. As noted earlier, soldiers trust each other with their lives, and the bonds they develop are very strong. Sexual assault of one soldier by another is an extreme violation of these bonds. The survivor's sense of trust can be shattered. Sheila had struggled with being one of a few women in a National Guard unit that was deployed to Afghanistan. She initially felt out of place. It seemed to her that all the men were watching her and waiting for her to fail. Over time, her hard work earned her the respect of her fellow soldiers, and her comfort and confidence grew. This changed abruptly, however, when 8 months into her deployment she was sexually assaulted by two soldiers from the base where she was stationed. After the assault, Sheila felt a profound sense of abandonment and loneliness. If she couldn't trust other American soldiers in a foreign country full of insurgents, whom could she rely on? Who had her back? When she returned to the States, she found it impossible to trust anyone. She had believed that her fellow soldiers would have risked their lives for her, yet they assaulted her. Civilians seemed even less trustworthy—what might they do to her?

As noted in Chapter 9, survivors of sexual assault may feel invalidated when others don't believe that the assault occurred or the legal system does not support them. Survivors of military sexual trauma can experience similar invalidation. Hank was raped by three other soldiers during a training exercise in his second year of service. Two weeks after the assault, he confided in a chaplain, who encouraged him to report the assault to his commanders. When he did, he was stunned that his unit commander, who had always told them they could come to him with anything, was skeptical. When an official complaint was made, the base leaders accused Hank of making up the story. The complaint was eventually quashed due to lack of evidence, even though Hank had identified his assailants. Like Sheila, he felt totally alone. He had volunteered to serve his country and sacrifice his life if need be, and these people were supposed to take care of him. Where were they when he needed them most? He came away from this experience believing that no matter what authority figures said, they would turn on him whenever they wanted. This led to struggles after his discharge and return to civilian life. Hank didn't feel safe in the workplace and didn't trust his supervisors, so he rarely complied with their instructions. As a result, he was fired from a string of jobs. His brother Zach had been puzzled by this because, prior to going into the service, Hank had always shown respect for authority and had been a reliable and diligent employee. It wasn't until Hank finally told him what had happened that Zach began to realize the changes in Hank hadn't come from nowhere.

Suicidal Thoughts and Behaviors

As we noted in Chapter 2, many trauma survivors have thoughts about hurting themselves or ending their lives. This also is true for service men and women who survive trauma. Rates of suicide among American service members have increased steadily over the years since the United States became involved in the wars in Iraq and Afghanistan.

Having PTSD increases risk for suicidal thoughts and suicide attempts, and depression and alcohol and drug abuse also increase the risk. If your loved one mentions wanting to die or talks about hurting or killing himself, don't ignore or dismiss him. Check in with him to see how serious he is. Your support is important, but if you are really concerned, don't try to handle the situation yourself. Those who get professional help are less likely to harm themselves. Encourage the survivor to talk to a medical provider, using the methods we discussed in Chapter 4 and the ones we talk about below. If you're concerned that dangerous behavior is imminent, call the police. Don't hesitate because you're concerned about embarrassing your loved one or violating a confidence. The most important thing is to keep him safe. If you're concerned that his life is at risk, everything else is secondary.

Unique Aspects of Serving in Iraq and Afghanistan

Although some aspects of war have been consistent since the beginning of written history, the wars in Iraq and Afghanistan present unique challenges for military personnel who have served there. Multiple deployments, more female soldiers, greater contact with family during deployment, higher rates of survival from injuries, and higher rates of traumatic brain injuries are all new to these conflicts.

Multiple Deployments

The conflicts in Iraq and Afghanistan are the first in which many members of the armed forces have experienced **multiple deployments**. Previously, American soldiers served a tour in the war zone and then returned home for good, often being discharged from the military. In past conflicts soldiers returned to the war zone only if they chose to do so.

The potential for future deployments can have enormous effects on readjustment. Some service members feel less motivated to resume their life activities after they return from deployment. They may think, "Why bother going back to work or starting school again if they can just send me back there?" Others simply never let their guard down between deployments and go about life as if they are still in the war zone. They remain watchful and on guard and highly reactive to perceived threat, sleeping poorly and limiting activities to maintain safety. Those between deployments may not seek treatment for trauma-related difficulties because they believe any treatment gains would be undone by future deployment.

Female Service Members

Although women have served their countries in the military in past wars, the current conflicts in Iraq and Afghanistan are the first time in American history that **women have served in the war zone** in large numbers. More than 10 percent of the soldiers deployed to Iraq and Afghanistan have been women, and they have contributed in countless ways to the military efforts in those wars. Although women still are not assigned to combat duties, they nonetheless have been subjected to serious dangers in these conflicts in unprecedented ways. This is because of the fact that there has been no real "front line" in Iraq and Afghanistan, and insurgents' violent activities are frequent and pervasive throughout the war zone. Women serving in Iraq and Afghanistan often are exposed to the same levels of threat and danger that their male comrades experience.

Many female service members feel extra pressure to excel at their duties so that the ability of all women to serve won't be questioned. When any of the guys in Gina's unit screwed up during training, they got a lot of ribbing from everyone. But when she or the other two women in the unit screwed up, they always heard things like "Oh, poor little girl!" or "Come on, honey, you gotta earn your place here!" After a while, Gina felt like she was taking the reputation of every woman in the military on her shoulders whenever she did anything, and this put immense pressure on her to succeed.

Another issue for female service members is that the transition back to parenting roles may be harder for them than it is for male service members. Paul felt like he had missed important milestones of his son's life while he was deployed. When Amelie deployed, she had been staying at home to care for her two children, who were 2 and 5. After 7 months in Afghanistan, she returned to the role of primary caretaker for the children, but felt like she was a babysitter or nanny. In the time she had been gone, her children seemed to have changed so much, and the younger one seemed at first to be a little scared of her. Amelie felt like she had lost her maternal bond with her children, and she didn't know whether she could ever get it back. She was devastated by this, and because she had always prided herself on being a strong woman, she beat herself up for being such a "wimp" about it.

Increased Contact Between Home and the War Zone

Developments in technology have increased the ease of **contact between home and the war zone.** In past wars, soldiers were limited to writing letters to communicate with family and friends at home. Military personnel deployed to Iraq or Afghanistan have been able to communicate with family and friends instantaneously via e-mail, cell phones, and webcams. This has helped families stay connected and eased the stress of being away from home. Webcams helped Aaron and Julie feel in touch with each other's daily lives during his lengthy deployments in Afghanistan. A webcam in the delivery room enabled Aaron to "be there" for Julie during the birth of their daughter. But in some cases such close contact has had negative effects. When Mark and Eva spoke each week, she shared with him how much his boys were struggling without him. He found that for the rest of the week thoughts of his sons distracted him from focusing on his duties in the war zone. At the beginning of her deployment, Maria had called Wallace once a week to check in and tell him how she was. This changed after a particularly bad firefight when Maria was faced with a large number of wounded personnel and she and her medical crew had to prioritize whom they would try to save. She couldn't bear to talk with Wallace that week, or the next. How could she tell him about that? It was hard enough for her to think about. The ease of communication made the difficult experience more complicated for Maria while she was still in the war zone. Back at home, Wallace was really worried by Maria's silence. What had happened to her? Was she okay?

Higher Rates of Survival from Serious Injuries

Troops deployed to Iraq and Afghanistan have experienced significant violence. The National Center for PTSD estimated that 80% of troops serving in Iraq in 2006 received incoming fire, and 60% were attacked or ambushed during their deployment. More than 60% reported seeing human remains, and most knew someone who was seriously injured or killed. Due to advances in protective equipment and medical technologies, many members of the armed forces are surviving severe injuries that previously would have been fatal. As a result, more American soldiers are coming home alive. Military, veteran, and civilian medical systems are caring for more injured soldiers, many with complex injuries and pain conditions that are difficult to treat. Many service members and veterans are struggling with the aftermath of those injuries, as well as the scars and pain that serve as reminders of horrific events. Coping with chronic pain is challenging in itself. Posttraumatic stress and pain problems together can create a cycle of pain, anxiety, and stress that is hard to break.

Traumatic Brain Injuries

Mark was driving a large truck in a long convoy of vehicles when an improvised explosive device was detonated under his vehicle. Mark and his passenger were both driven upward by the blast, and Mark, who was a few inches taller, hit his head on the roof of the cab. He was woozy for the next few moments and afterward didn't have a clear memory of how the convoy was stopped and he and his passenger were removed from the vehicle. Later, when he was more "with it," his buddies kidded him about having gotten his "bell rung" by the blast. He had a headache for a couple of days after that, and sometimes got dizzy.

Many soldiers deployed to Iraq and Afghanistan experienced explosions that can result in brain injury. In fact, those injured in Iraq and Afghanistan are twice as likely to have had a brain injury as those injured in the Vietnam war. The effects of brain injuries can vary widely. For most soldiers, the injuries are mild and they will be back to normal within a few months. Those who experience more severe injuries, however, may develop longer-lasting symptoms such as poor concentration, impulsive behavior, memory problems, irritability, visual or hearing impairments, sensitivity to light or noise, headaches, sleep problems, anxiety, and depression. When they are caused by a head injury, these symptoms are known collectively as *postconcussive syndrome*.

Due to the overlap in symptoms, brain injury can complicate the assessment and treatment of posttraumatic stress. Soldiers who have been in combat are at higher risk for both brain injury and PTSD. It sometimes can be difficult to determine the cause of symptoms like irritability, poor sleep, and difficulty concentrating. Military personnel and veterans deployed to Iraq or Afghanistan are screened for exposure to events that may have resulted in a brain injury upon their return. Often, returning warriors will focus on the head injury as the cause of such symptoms and downplay the role of posttraumatic stress. Posttraumatic stress is common among those with postconcussive syndrome, however, and treatment of posttraumatic stress can alleviate many of the symptoms attributed to the brain injury. Moreover, treatments for posttraumatic symptoms are just as effective for warriors who have suffered brain injuries as for those who have not. Also, there are specific interventions to help with postconcussive symptoms that, together with treatment of posttraumatic stress and depression, can result in major improvements.

Treatment after Military Trauma

The fact that war affects those who wage it has been written about since the days of ancient Greece. But PTSD did not exist as a formal mental health diagnosis until 1980. In the early 1990s, during the time of the first Gulf War, PTSD was well documented and researched, but treatments were still being developed. Advances in treatment research over the last 15 years have led to the effective treatments described in Chapter 4. The wars in Iraq and Afghanistan were the first time the United States went to war prepared with knowledge of how to treat PTSD. Significant efforts have been made to make these treatments widely available to military personnel and veterans suffering the aftereffects of war.

As we noted earlier, military trauma is associated with many of the same aftereffects as civilian trauma, plus the specific challenges of readjustment following deployment and return to civilian life. The same is true for treatment. The treatment issues we discussed in Chapters 3 and 4, including the barriers and the potential positive outcomes, apply to treatment for military trauma. Available evidence indicates that trauma-focused CBT can be helpful for military personnel and veterans suffering posttraumatic symptoms. Earlier research had found that military populations did not benefit from treatment as much as civilians. The lesser response to treatment may be due to the era and conflicts in which the survivors served, complicating aspects of readjustment, and the array of physical and mental health problems that war survivors face. In formulating a treatment plan, a good therapist will take time to consider the various problems affecting your loved one, including difficulties with readjustment as well as other clinical problems.

Service members and veterans face unique obstacles, and their treatment can be affected by a number of variables. Fortunately, in the United States there are specialized programs to address these specific needs in military hospitals, Veterans Affairs medical centers, and Vet Centers. We will describe treatment options and then we'll talk about how your loved one can overcome obstacles and benefit from available help.

Treatment from Military Providers

Increased awareness of PTSD and the availability of treatment have led to unprecedented efforts by the U.S. Department of Defense to address the psychological needs of active-duty soldiers. Starting in 2006, the Department of Defense and the Department of Veterans Affairs began training large numbers of health care providers in the state-of-the-art treatments for PTSD and depression discussed in Chapter 4. Military behavioral health clinicians are better equipped than ever before to treat the range of problems that might interfere with service members performing their duties. In addition, behavioral health clinicians often are available in the war zone to assess and treat problems as they arise.

VA Medical Centers and Community-Based Outpatient Clinics

Veterans who received honorable or general discharges and who either have conditions that have been judged to be connected to military service or meet certain income criteria are eligible for care through the Department of Veterans Affairs, generally known as the VA. Members of the National Guard and of any branch of the reserves also are eligible if they were activated, served honorably, and meet the income or service connection requirements.

Veterans returning from the conflicts in Afghanistan and Iraq are entitled to five years of free services for any problems related to their combat deployment. When he came back, Darren received physical rehabilitation to learn how to use the remaining fingers on his left hand more effectively and also was fitted for two different kinds of prosthetics. He received this care free of charge because his injury occurred in the course of his combat deployment. Also, if a veteran has a medical condition that has been documented to be due to any aspect of his military service, medical care for that condition is provided free of charge. Depending on how much the service-connected condition interferes with the veteran's functioning, he also may receive other care and medication free of charge. Veterans whose income falls below a certain level can receive VA care free of charge. Also, veterans are not charged for treatment of any condition resulting from military sexual trauma. It took Sheila several years to go to the VA for help with the posttraumatic symptoms caused by the sexual assault she suffered while on active duty. When she did, she was relieved to find out that the treatment would not cost her anything.

VA medical centers provide a wide range of medical and mental health services. In addition, smaller community-based outpatient clinics offer primary medical care and some mental health treatment to veterans who live far from a VA medical center. There are VA medical centers or community-based outpatient clinics in every state in the United States, as well as in Guam, Puerto Rico, American Samoa, and the Virgin Islands. Contact information is included in the Resources section at the back of the book.

One of the advantages of VA care is that, except for some services provided to spouses and family members, VA staff work only with veterans. Many VA medical and mental health providers are trained in VA internships or residencies. Although many VA staff did not serve in the military, they all are very familiar with the specific concerns of veterans. Most VA providers are aware of the potential problems that the process of readjusting to civilian life can cause your loved one, and they will be able to integrate these problems into the treatment plan. Also, all the various VA providers keep a single electronic medical record, accessible anywhere within the VA system. George, who served in Vietnam, had been receiving his medical care through the VA system in Vermont. He finally opened up to his primary care doctor about the nightmares that had plagued him off and on for years. His doctor immediately referred him to the mental health service. Soon, George had an appointment with a psychiatrist, who talked with him about medication options. His psychiatrist checked his medical record and assured George that the medications he was taking for blood pressure and prostate problems would not interfere with treatment. He also referred George to a psychologist, who discussed nonpharmacological treatment options. The "one-stop shopping" VA medical centers often provide results in higher-quality care than treatment by several independent practitioners.

The VA is the largest integrated health care system in the United States. Although there are many staff offering many services in many medical centers, the system prides itself on operating as "one VA." When George and his wife, Mindy, retired from Vermont to Florida, Mindy was worried that George, who was receiving all of his care from the VA, would have to go through a lot of red tape at the new medical center that would delay his prescription renewals. His doctors in Vermont assured him this would not be the case. A week after they arrived in Florida, she and George went to the nearest VA medical center. Within a few hours he was registered and had a medical appointment. When George met with his new doctor, she already knew his medical history, right down to where he had served in Vietnam. After taking time to get to know him and doing an exam, she renewed his prescriptions.

The U.S. Department of Veterans Affairs Health Administration is always working to ensure that returning soldiers and veterans of all eras have access to the highest-quality health care possible. In many areas, the VA provides the most advanced, state-of-the-art care available. This is the case for PTSD treatment. The massive national training program mentioned earlier has made the latest evidence-based therapies for PTSD, depression, and related problems available through VA clinicians who understand the specific issues facing veterans.

Vet Centers

As hard as she tried, Polly just couldn't convince Frank to go to the VA. He always reminded her that he had already tried to get help at a VA hospital in the mid-1970s. But when they told him there was nothing wrong with him, he had vowed never to set foot in a VA facility again. Polly watched him try several community therapists who simply didn't understand enough about what veterans go through to be helpful. One day while browsing on the VA's website, Polly saw a link for something called "Vet Centers." Intrigued, she spent the afternoon researching and reading.

In the late 1970s, the government realized that Vietnam veterans were struggling to readjust to civilian life. At this time, VA medical centers were not well equipped to provide outpatient therapy for PTSD—remember, PTSD didn't become recognized as a diagnosis until 1980. Due to the draft, the negative politics of the war, and negative homecoming experiences, Vietnam veterans were particularly mistrusting of the government. As a result, many Vietnam veterans did not feel comfortable turning to large government-run medical centers for help. Also, Vietnam veterans, due to their extreme sense of disconnection from civilians, were uncomfortable receiving counseling from the mostly civilian VA therapy staff. As a result, the government established Vet Centers—small, freestanding community centers staffed by veterans and designed to be more welcoming. Unlike the much larger VA medical centers, Vet Centers do not provide medical care. They focus entirely on counseling for readjustment after war or other military stressors. Most Vet Center staff are themselves veterans and are very familiar with the issues surrounding military service and understand the specific ways that trauma can affect those who have served.

Since their early days, the scope of service of Vet Centers has expanded. Currently, they provide free services to all veterans who were deployed to war zones or peacekeeping missions as well as to survivors of military sexual trauma. Available services usually include individual and group treatment, couple counseling, and family therapy. Family members of veterans who are eligible to receive services at Vet Centers also can receive certain services free of charge, as can the surviving families of service members who die while on active duty. Vet Centers are federal facilities, but they keep separate records from VA medical centers, so veterans who do not want their counseling records seen by VA staff can preserve their confidentiality.

State and Local Programs

Although service members and veterans may be eligible for military or VA medical services, they are not obliged to use those services. Many states have their own departments of veterans affairs and offer services to veterans to complement what the national VAs provide. Some states offer veterans free health care in their community facilities. Others contract with local mental health professionals so that veterans can receive care free of charge where they live. Some veterans find state services appealing because their health care information is not stored in the federal government's database. In fact, some states specifically offer services that cannot be connected to the veteran's VA or military records.

Community Providers

Service members and veterans also may opt to seek treatment from therapists in the community who are skilled in the treatment of post-traumatic problems. The Department of Defense sometimes contracts with civilian providers to provide services to active-duty soldiers. For some veterans who live a very long distance from the closest VA facility, the VA contracts with civilian providers for care closer to home. In other cases, service members and veterans seek care from civilian providers when they are not comfortable receiving services from the federal government. Most civilian providers do not know as much about the military as does the Department of Defense, VA, or Vet Center staff. They may not be familiar with the process of readjustment that returning service members go through. Yet they may be just as skilled at delivering evidence-based therapies for PTSD.

Zach's brother Hank had planned on making a career out of the Army, but this changed after he was sexually assaulted. When leadership didn't support his complaint, it seemed like the whole Army had turned its back on him after he had been ready to commit his life to the service. After he was discharged, Hank wanted no contact with the military, the VA, or the government. Zach knew that VAs and Vet Centers both provided free treatment for survivors of military sexual trauma, but Hank would have nothing to do with them. So Zach went to the counseling center at his college and asked whether they knew of any local providers who specialized in treating rape survivors. He walked out with a list of three psychologists and two social workers. Hank settled on one of the social workers and started therapy with her. Although he had to explain a lot about the Army to his therapist, he was glad there was no connection to the military or the government.

Obstacles to Getting Help

Although you may be glad to know that your loved one has more treatment options because of his military service, it may be frustrating to learn that he faces additional barriers to therapy. We'll discuss these barriers and what you can do to help your loved one surmount them.

The Biggest Obstacle: Stigma

The stigma associated with mental illness is a tremendous barrier to seeking help. Many people feel ashamed of their emotional struggles because they think that mental health problems indicate something negative about the person suffering them. People diagnosed with psychiatric conditions often are labeled with pejorative terms such as "crazy," "nuts," "psycho," or "loony." They are seen as weak, unstable, dangerous, and unable to live among "normal" people. Others may not trust them with daily tasks or may exclude them from activities that they fear might "stress" them and cause a "breakdown." People with mental illnesses are deemed unfit to hold high-level jobs or engage in intense or demanding activities. These beliefs have been present in various cultures for hundreds of years, and, like many other prejudicial beliefs that human beings hold, they are the result of ignorance and fear. Unfortunately, those prejudices are very real, and they can deter those suffering from mental health difficulties from seeking help and disclosing their problems to others.

This stigma associated with psychiatric diagnoses has been very apparent to us in our work with trauma survivors. We have seen patients suffer quietly with treatable conditions for many years, simply because they were afraid to tell anyone they were having problems. Often, during the first session, such patients acknowledge that although they were embarrassed to share what was bothering them, they felt good finally getting it off their chests.

A variety of factors specific to military culture intensify the power of stigma for warriors and veterans. First and foremost is the value that military culture places on physical and emotional strength. Soldiers are trained to do their jobs even if they are suffering or in pain. They learn to push their discomfort aside and accomplish the mission no matter what they must endure. When confronted with a life-or-death situation, this ability to push on in the face of adversity is extremely valuable. Soldiers do not stop trying. An unfortunate consequence of this resistance to pain, however, is that soldiers can be reluctant to acknowledge that there is a problem and to get help for it. A soldier who repeatedly hears, "You feel no pain, you never give up," can find it hard to admit any injury, be it physical or psychological. Mental injury, in particular, is perceived as a sign of weakness, because a warrior is strong above all else.

Paul had started having bad dreams while he was still in Iraq. Even his fellow Marines seemed slightly uncomfortable with how tense and on edge he was all the time. When they were sent back to the States, most of the other guys seemed to relax, but not Paul. He barely slept, and he always seemed ready for a fight. After 3 months, his sergeant finally sat Paul down and told him he was worried about him. "Son, other Marines can handle you, but civilians can't. I'm concerned that you're going to do something bad to someone who has no idea what they're messing with," his gunny said. "I think it's time you tried to get some help." Paul had no idea what to make of what he had been told. *Help?* What did *that* mean? The guys in Paul's platoon had always made fun of people who needed "help," either physically or mentally. If you complained, you were broken, or weak, or a "wuss."

Fear of stigma is exacerbated by the fact that it's difficult to keep secrets in the military. As a member of a small, tight unit, a soldier who reports that she is having problems risks everyone else finding out. After Gina's National Guard unit came back from Afghanistan, she couldn't bear attending the monthly trainings. Seeing weapons, military vehicles, and other soldiers brought back bad memories of the ambush, and she couldn't stand the pain. The Saturday night of the first monthly training, two separate fellow Guard members called her asking what the problem was. Their sergeant had refused to tell them what was wrong with her, so they both assumed it was something "mental." Why else wouldn't he tell them the problem? Gina couldn't believe that it had taken them less than 24 hours to figure out that she was having difficulties. Paul knew that if he went to the behavioral health staff on base, everyone would find out and he would never hear the end of it. Paul decided to keep his problems to himself to avoid the judgments of other Marines.

For some, the stereotypes associated with "combat veterans" can lead to reluctance to seek help. Marcus had grown up watching the same movies about the aftermath of the Vietnam War that everyone else had seen, and he was aware of the stereotype of the "crazy Vietnam veteran." He didn't want people to think he was "shell-shocked" or violent, so he tried not to talk about the difficulties he was having. George, who had served honorably in Vietnam, had worked with people over the years who had made remarks like "Don't get George mad at you; he was in Vietnam! He might go crazy!" After hearing comments like these for years, George himself had begun to believe that if he went to a mental health provider for help, it would mean that the things those people had said were true and he really was crazy.

The main thing you can do to help your loved one overcome the stigma associated with seeking mental health treatment is to identify your own prejudices and work hard to change them. Practice a supportive and nonjudgmental stance toward your loved one and his problems. If he perceives that you are not judging him because of his emotional reactions, then he will feel supported and may be less judgmental of himself. And he may be able to see the prejudices of others as ignorant beliefs and not facts. When Paul got home, he stayed quiet about the problems he was having, but his father, Ken, finally confronted him after he found Paul hiding in the basement during a big family gathering for a child's birthday. Paul was initially evasive but finally came clean to his father about the anger, the tension, and the nightmares about shooting the child in Iraq. Ken found himself wondering, as Paul was talking, whether Paul was one of those "crazy vets" who were going to "go postal" in the supermarket or the town hall. But Ken kept reminding himself that this was his son and that Paul was not "crazy," just struggling with coming home from war. Ken was able to tell Paul that the things he was experiencing were understandable reactions to war and that there were people who could help him. Paul had been terrified of disclosing his difficulties because he thought he would be "locked up." He felt like a huge burden had been lifted from him. By being aware of his own beliefs about mental illness, Ken was able to put his prejudices aside and support his son, who in turn felt like he wasn't so "broken" after all.

Fear of Negative Effects

Soldiers are often concerned about the negative effects that psychiatric treatment might have on their careers. This is due in part to the stigma and in part to uncertainty over the confidentiality of medical records. Chet had been with the National Guard for 12 years before his deployment to Iraq. He had been activated numerous times in his own state to help out during hurricanes and bad snowstorms, and he was proud of his work with the Guard. The Iraq deployment was really hard for him, though, mostly because of the deaths of two men who had been in the Guard with him from the beginning. They were killed by a bomb, and Chet had been charged with the awful task of gathering up their remains. He had felt detached from the whole thing while he was in Iraq and focused on getting through each day. But after he came home, he was having bizarre nightmares involving body parts of his friends and the grim reaper. He often woke up in a cold sweat, thrashing and yelling. He was so tired during the day he could barely do his job, and he was no fun to be around. His wife, Robinne, kept begging him to tell his superiors. He knew he needed help, but he wanted to serve 20 years in the Guard. What would happen if they knew he was screwed up? Would his whole career go down the drain?

Robinne had attended a postdeployment event with Chet and the other Guard families in his unit, and she had heard unit leadership clearly say that they really wanted soldiers to get help if they needed it. When Robinne tried to remind Chet of this and encourage him to ask for help, he shook his head. "You don't hear the jokes and the laughing," he told her. Chet explained that the same leaders who spoke at the event cracked jokes and belittled soldiers who were struggling either physically or psychologically. Although Chet knew other soldiers who had sought help and were still in the Guard, he feared he would be kicked out.

Service members and veterans also may be concerned about who can see their records. It is important to remember that when a citizen enlists with any branch of the armed forces he basically signs himself over to the care of the military. Service members and veterans often believe that anyone in the military can view their records without their consent, and in some cases this is true. When, after almost a year struggling on his own, Chet finally decided to seek help, he went to a private clinician in his town. At the first visit he asked the social worker what he would document, and, "Who's gonna read this?" When the social worker explained that he had no relationship with the government, Chet didn't really believe him. Chet started therapy but found it very difficult to open up about what was bothering him. He was "receiving treatment" but was holding back the main problems he was experiencing because he didn't trust his therapist. This avoidance interfered with therapy and prevented Chet from benefiting fully.

Are these concerns realistic? We have seen a very wide range of leadership responses to soldiers in need of help. While the military is working hard to create a climate that is conducive to help-seeking, change of this nature comes slowly. Fortunately, many leaders have been supportive of their soldiers seeking and receiving treatment so that they can continue to perform their duties at a high level. This is not universally the case, however, so it's difficult to predict what your loved one might experience.

You may be confused by the reluctance of the soldier or veteran in your life to seek treatment from either her military unit or the VA. Be aware of the concerns she might have about confidentiality and the potential for negative consequences for her career. Current service members and veterans should ask prospective treatment providers what they will document in their records and who will be able to read those records. Support the trauma survivor in your life, but remember that ultimately it is her decision, and if she is unwilling to use military or VA services, then it may be best to help her find alternatives that she believes are safer.

Young Veterans and the VA

When Jenny went with Marcus to one of his postdeployment functions, she heard representatives from the local VA talk about the care available to combat veterans. There were even computers set up to register the soldiers in the VA system right then and there. This had sounded like a good idea, but whenever Jenny mentioned going to the VA, Marcus shook his head. "VAs are full of old veterans," he would say. "Guys go in there and never come out. The VA's scary!" Jenny didn't believe him, and kept asking him about it, but Marcus kept refusing. Things kept getting worse, and about a year after he came back, Marcus finally agreed to go in and talk to someone. When they walked through the front door of the large VA medical center in their city, Jenny's worst fears were realized—all they could see were older men, some in wheelchairs, sitting in the main lobby. She held her breath, but Marcus kept going and walked to the registration desk.

When he identified himself as a returning Iraq veteran who wanted to register for services, the employee smiled and told Marcus she was glad he had come in. She took all of his information and spent almost a half-hour talking to him about all the benefits to which he was entitled (half of which neither Jenny nor Marcus had heard about). While she spoke, Jenny looked around, and she started to notice more and more younger veterans walking through the main lobby for appointments. The registration clerk gave Marcus a primary care appointment and told him that his doctor would coordinate any other care he needed. On their way out of the lobby, a few older veterans stopped Marcus and asked whether he had just gotten home. When he said he had been in Iraq, they shook his hand, thanked him, and kept saying, "Welcome home." It seemed to Jenny that, unlike the discomfort Marcus felt when friends said those things to him, he seemed genuinely appreciative of the kind words from the other veterans. Out in the parking lot, Jenny asked him why this was. Marcus smiled at her and said, "It's different coming from them. They know."

A larger number of American soldiers served in World War II, the Korean War, and Vietnam than the number of soldiers who have served since then. As a result, the veteran population in America has steadily become older—most veterans served by the VA were born in the 1950s or earlier. This can be a positive factor for veterans of those eras. When Roger retired at age 65, memories of his time in Vietnam started bothering him more and more. He decided that the VA would be a good option for his health care because changes in his health insurance limited his access to other providers. At his first primary care visit, the physician's assistant recommended that he see a mental health provider for help with the painful memories and nightmares. He was soon referred to a PTSD group and was surprised to find that it was mostly Vietnam veterans, one of whom, it turned out, had been in Phu Bai around the same time as Roger. After having felt isolated for so many years, Roger felt more at home with the group than he had with anyone in a long time. He knew that they had been through what he had been through, and they understood.

For younger veterans like Marcus, the older age of the veteran population can make the VA seem less comfortable. However, as more and more soldiers deploy to and then return from Iraq and Afghanistan, more young veterans are electing to receive their medical care at the VA. Some VAs have even established treatment programs specifically for younger veterans. Like many hospitals offering a full range of services, VA medical centers can seem large, intimidating, and hard to navigate. If the veteran in your life is considering getting care at the VA, it can help to spend some time at the closest medical center talking to the staff at the information desk. Your loved one can find out what services are available and for which she is eligible. Every VA medical center has at least one staff person dedicated to ensuring that veterans who served in Iraq and Afghanistan get the care they need as soon as possible. Usually this person's name and picture are posted through-out the medical center. If the trauma survivor in your life served in Operation Iraqi Freedom or Enduring Freedom, finding the OEF/OIF Program Manager at the closest VA medical center would be the best way to start receiving care at the VA.

Service Connection and Benefits

Earlier, we mentioned that veterans could receive free care from the VA for any injury or condition that resulted from their military service. The Veterans Benefits Administration, or VBA, accepts claims from vet-erans that a medical or psychological condition was caused by service in the military, or is *service connected*. While he was overseas, Aaron developed a rash on his stomach. The rash never quite went away dur-ing his deployment or for about a year afterward. At that time he sub-mitted a claim that the rash was due to his deployment. To evaluate his claim, a physician conducted a medical examination that included a detailed history and physical exam.

There are two steps to evaluating a service-connection claim. First, the VBA decides whether the veteran's military service caused his condition. Second, the VBA determines how much that condition affects the veteran's life. Some conditions, such as scars, may not sig-nificantly affect the veteran's functioning; they may not prevent the veteran from working or doing the things that he likes to do. Other, more debilitating conditions, such as the loss of a leg, blindness, or severe depression, may have a much greater impact, making it difficult for the veteran to engage in hobbies, develop relationships, or keep a job. If the service-connected condition is judged to interfere with the veteran's functioning, the veteran receives monetary compensation for the lost functioning as well as some additional benefits. The greater the impairment, the more money the veteran receives.

This can be a confusing situation for some veterans. On the one hand, they want very much to get better. On the other hand, they may lose money and some benefits if they get better. Research into the relationship between service connection and treatment has shown that it's complex. It is generally agreed, however, that receiving money in exchange for being disabled may interfere with the treatment and recovery process.

Strength and Support: What You Can Do

The service member or veteran in your life may face unique challenges, but he also will have more sources of support and help. Although we have described many different problems that can complicate your loved one's situation and various treatment options, the tips and recommendations we made in Chapters 3–8 will be just as helpful for you. We recommend that you research the treatment options available to you and your loved one as much as possible, so that you both know what opportunities exist for change. Once you and your loved one have learned about the treatment options available, you can use the pro–con analysis from Chapter 3 to help you decide which one might be best, and you can ask potential therapists the questions we listed in Chapter 5 to refine your decision. We recommend that you employ the tips for self-care that we discussed in Chapter 6 to help you cope with the additional complications faced by survivors of military trauma. If you're trying to determine how long you're willing to wait for your loved one to address his symptoms and reintegrate into the civilian world, we recommend you consult Chapter 7 to help you decide where you're willing to set your limits and then use the tips for assertiveness in Chapter 8 to convey this to your loved one. The problems facing your loved one are more complex due to his military service, but the same methods can help you take care of yourself and support your loved one.

We also recommend that you remind yourself as much as possible of the context in which your loved one's trauma took place. The survivor in your life was traumatized while serving his country. He was willing to put himself on the line for the rest of us, and for that he deserves respect and support. Also, remembering that he is a soldier or veteran can remind you of his many strengths. As we noted earlier, soldiers are trained to endure great pain to complete their mission. If through support and help your loved one can focus that great strength and endurance on recovery, he has an excellent chance of living a happy, healthy life.

PART IV

Putting Your Lives Back Together

ELEVEN

Reconnecting with Your Partner and Helping Your Children

The night she learned Jim was burned in the fire at the factory was one of the worst nights of Connie's life. She slept at the hospital that night and the next, waiting for word on Jim's condition. She was horrified to see Jim in so much pain—the whole right side of his arm was burned, and the doctors said he was going to need skin grafts but that he would be okay. It was hard to watch him struggle with the pain. But the worst part was that he didn't want to talk about what happened. She knew he had tried to help one of his coworkers who ended up on the burn unit for months, but he refused to tell her anything. And in the months that followed, she felt like he was slipping away from her—he seemed so distant. Whereas he used to be sociable, now he was becoming a recluse. Life returned to normal, but Jim did not. He went back to work, but he no longer got together with his buddies from work for poker night. When he came home, he just ate, watched TV, and went to bed long before their usual bedtime. They no longer went for their after-dinner walks, and laughter was a thing of the past. It seemed like the spark was gone and he no longer cared about being close with her.

Meagan felt stuck. Before Charlie had deployed to Afghanistan, Meagan had thought he was "the one" and they would get married and settle down. But after he got back, it seemed like they had no emotional connection anymore. He kept to himself and was moody all the time. No matter what she tried, she couldn't figure out how to communicate with him. And their sex life was completely different. Before he left, he was always pestering her to have sex, and she practically had to shoo him away at times. But after his deployment, he seemed much less interested in being intimate and even stopped her on a few occasions when she tried to initiate sex, which had never happened before. And when they did have sex, it felt like an act, like they weren't connected at all. Charlie was always a typical guy and had never been fond of snuggling or cuddling, but now it didn't even feel like they were people anymore when they had sex. To Meagan, it felt like they were robots. Although she knew she hadn't changed much since he left for Afghanistan, she started to wonder whether she just wasn't as attractive now. What was it that she wasn't giving him? After all the time they had been together, when it seemed like they were going to get married, how could she think about leaving him now?

No matter what Eli tried, he couldn't figure out how to talk to Marissa. It seemed like she had never really calmed down after the hurricane. She was always either completely withdrawn or really angry, and he never knew which he would get. Once his tiny little wife had actually thrown a phone at him in a fit of rage and then immediately retreated into the basement for the night. No matter how gentle or kind he was, she could still snap for no reason at all. What really confused him was that at times it seemed like she wanted him to talk to her, like she wanted him to tell her that she would be okay or that there was nothing to be afraid of, but he had no idea what to say or how to help her.

The effects of trauma can extend far outward, touching those around the survivor. If you are in a close relationship with a trauma survivor with PTSD, you may be experiencing the devastating effects that trauma can have on a relationship. Living with a trauma survivor with PTSD can be stressful. You might be feeling tense, anxious, depressed, lonely, confused, and even guilty. The changes in your lives can feel like a burden, and you may feel worn out by day-to-day life. On the whole, if you are like many partners of trauma survivors suffering posttraumatic reactions, you may be feeling dissatisfied with your relationship; you may even be questioning your commitment to "sticking it out." In this chapter we discuss how posttraumatic reactions affect those in intimate relationships with the trauma survivor. We'll look at what is known about how relationships are affected and what can be done to repair them. A lot less is known about how a survivor's posttraumatic stress may affect children in the family, but we offer some insights and advice for helping them as well. You also may find that our discussion of closeness and connection applies to children as well as to your individual relationship with the survivor.

How Relationships Can Be Affected by Trauma

Intimate relationships of trauma survivors can be affected in a variety of ways. Some trauma survivors have so much difficulty establishing close interpersonal relationships that they never marry. In many cases, however, survivors were in intimate relationships before the traumatic event or before the onset or worsening of PTSD or other problems. Also, many survivors *do* enter into relationships in spite of their difficulties, and problems maintaining a close connection with their partners emerge when the relationship is well under way. If you are struggling in your relationship with a trauma survivor, your situation may be one of the latter two scenarios.

The issues affecting relationships are readily apparent for some groups of trauma survivors. For example, it's easy to see why survivors of domestic violence might have difficulties trusting their partners or how survivors of sexual assault might have difficulties with sexual intimacy. But it's less obvious how other types of trauma might affect relationships. In 1978 the President's Commission on Mental Health reported that nearly 40% of Vietnam veterans' marriages dissolved within 6 months of returning from the war zone. These statistics were startling, and they spawned a flurry of research into the effects of war trauma on the marriages of military veterans. Since that time, we have learned a lot more about how trauma can damage a marriage and lead to divorce. In particular, we know that the effects of trauma on relationships are due largely to symptoms of posttraumatic stress, not to anything about traumatic events themselves, so the relationships of survivors of all types of trauma can be impaired. Although much of what we know about the effects of trauma on intimate relationships has come from studies of the marriages of male veterans, most of this work applies equally to the intimate relationships of other trauma survivors suffering PTSD. There are some ways that relationships of survivors of other types of trauma are affected that are not evident from the work on military families that we address along the way.

PTSD Can Devastate Relationships

As we noted earlier, a consistent finding from research on trauma survivors' intimate relationships is that most of the effects of trauma on relationships are caused by PTSD symptoms, even at low levels. In other words, it is not the experience of trauma per se, but rather posttraumatic reactions that negatively affect relationships. Emotional numbing and interpersonal withdrawal contribute much to the disconnection between partners. Trauma survivors' nightmares can affect their partners' sleep, leaving them irritable and fatigued. Hyperarousal symptoms also can affect partners. You may have noticed that after living with the survivor's fear and vigilance for so long, you have begun to adopt his anxious ways. Anger and irritability can lead to conflict, hostility, and verbal abuse toward the partner and in some instances this escalates to physical violence.

The negative effects of PTSD on relationships have been observed in veterans of different wars (World War II, Vietnam, and Iraq and Afghanistan) and different countries (the United States, Israel, New Zealand, and the Netherlands). The disruption can be substantial. Relationships of veterans with PTSD are two to three times as likely to be in distress as those without PTSD. We see similar patterns in the general population of the United States. People with PTSD are three to six times more likely to divorce as those without the diagnosis.

Veterans with PTSD tend to be lonely and unhappy with their relationships, but they are not alone in their misery—the breakdown of intimacy is felt on both sides of the relationship. Compared to spouses of combat veterans without PTSD, spouses of veterans with PTSD tend to report more symptoms of anxiety and depression as well as more health-related problems. They report less intimacy, more conflict, less satisfaction with their marriages, and less cohesion in their family relationships. Spouses of veterans with PTSD are less satisfied with sexual intimacy in their marriages, and they also report impairments in relationships outside their family. Finally, they report being less happy and less satisfied with their lives overall. What's important is that the extent of distress and marital dissatisfaction has been shown to be *related directly to the severity of the veteran's PTSD symptoms.* Moreover, without treatment, the negative effects of PTSD on marital satisfaction and the emotional well-being of the survivor and his partner are likely to endure for many years.

The negative effect of PTSD on families has led to a burgeoning area of research into the interpersonal aspects of trauma. More research has been conducted on this subject in the last 10 years than ever before, and we are starting to form a coherent picture of how relationships are affected by trauma. It is becoming clear from this research that partners have a critical role in trauma survivors' adaptation to trauma and that there are significant benefits to involving them in the treatment process. Considerable effort is being devoted to developing interventions to help families in distress enhance their intimacy and well-being. We return to this later, but first, let's look more closely at the ways that intimate relationships can be affected by PTSD.

Emotional Numbing, Withdrawal, and Restricted Communication

The trauma survivor's emotional withdrawal and isolation from you are the posttraumatic symptoms that can be most damaging to your relationship. This is because emotional involvement with one's partner has been shown to be critically important to the quality of the intimate relationship. The trauma survivor's emotional experience of love and happiness might be blunted. He might struggle to communicate his emotions openly and limit expressions of affection. To avoid provoking emotions related to the trauma, the survivor may not disclose much about his traumatic experience to you. Poor communication of emotion, affection, and the details of pivotal life experiences can erode the intimacy in your relationship. The survivor may feel that you and others cannot understand or relate to his experience, which makes him feel disconnected. The more he feels disconnected, the more he may detach from you and others in his life.

The survivor's efforts to avoid reminders of the trauma may be confusing to you and can lead to the survivor's spending increasing time alone, away from you and the family. He may withdraw from routine daily activities, visiting with friends, or participating in the lives of his children. His lack of communication, combined with seemingly bizarre behaviors such as flashbacks, vigilance, and anger outbursts, can lead to a further sense of his disconnection from your life. Emotional and behavioral withdrawal erodes communication and trust in family relationships and leads to further discord. The result is a recurring pattern of detachment, isolation, conflict, and withdrawal.

Ambiguous Loss

Ambiguous loss is a term used to describe any situation in which a loved one is absent in some ways but present in others. A family can be affected by ambiguous loss when the loved one is still a strong emotional presence in their lives but physically is absent. This can occur when family members are uncertain of the status of their loved one, such as when he is missing. The absence of conclusive information about the loved one prevents the family from making decisions and moving on with their lives and keeps them stuck in a sort of emotional limbo. Ambiguous loss also can affect a family when their loved one is physically present but emotionally or psychologically distant and not participating in family life. In her study of the families of Israeli war veterans, researcher Rachel Dekel has observed that family members of trauma survivors with PTSD often suffer from ambiguous loss. Although the trauma survivor is physically present in the family, he may be considered psychologically absent because he does not function as part of the family. The lack of clarity in the survivor's presence can leave the spouse immobilized with regard to decision making. This can lead to depression, anxiety, and guilt.

Caregiver Burden

When the survivor is not functioning in his usual life roles, often the partner takes over more responsibilities within the family, as well as the additional role of "caregiver." The spouse may take on primary responsibility for financially supporting the family. She may have more duties related to maintaining the household and taking care of children. The activities of taking care of her husband may include looking after his emotional as well as medical needs. Sometimes the survivor's level of fear and distress is so great that he becomes dependent on his spouse to meet his basic practical and emotional needs. This can be the case particularly when the survivor is struggling with physical injuries in addition to emotional stress. In such instances, the spouse may experience **caregiver burden**. After the fire, Jim required substantial medical care to restore functioning to his severely burned right arm. Connie had to change his bandages daily and assist him with bathing and dressing. And because he was right-handed, he was unable to write or perform many routine tasks. She was okay with all this in the beginning. But a year later, she was still spending all of her time taking him to appointments and taking care of daily living, and she felt so alone. She was starting to feel at her wits' end.

If your partner has become physically or emotionally dependent on you, you may feel like your relationship has become more like one of parent and child than of partners. You may begin to feel that the activities of caring for him as well as the household and children leave you little time for yourself. You may feel constantly busy and exhausted, and it can seem that you have lost your independence and sources of pleasure in life. Many partners of trauma survivors feel they have sacrificed much of what is important to them personally, socially, and financially for their partner. More severe PTSD symptoms and impairment in the survivor's daily life can lead to a greater sense of caregiver burden, which in turn can increase the partner's level of emotional distress and dissatisfaction with her marriage.

PTSD as a Contagious Condition

Researchers have noted that partners and family of trauma survivors sometimes also show signs of anxiety, depression, and even PTSD. This is sometimes referred to as **"secondary trauma."** Partners of trauma survivors with PTSD report higher levels of depression, anxiety, sleep difficulties, and stress-related health problems. Of course, in some instances, the partners themselves also may be trauma survivors. But what we are talking about here is not the effects of trauma in your life, but rather the stress of living with a trauma survivor. Researchers have noted that some partners of trauma survivors report that they gradually take on some of the symptoms that their partner experiences, as if PTSD were a contagious disease. For example, they may start to be more on guard for danger and may feel "keyed up" even when there's no real need to be. They may feel irritable and "snappy," and they can have trouble concentrating. They may sleep poorly and may even report disturbing dreams. Some say that they live their lives as if they are on the verge of a possible disaster, that they fear that their traumatized spouse might have a heart attack or stroke or commit suicide. Partners often feel irritated by the survivors' dependency on them. When the survivor is functioning in their relationship as if he is another child rather than a partner, the partner feels an absence of support. Partners may feel a loss of control over their lives and sometimes blame themselves for the difficulties they are having coping with the stress. Whether the emotional distress of trauma survivors' partners actually reflects a form of "vicarious PTSD" is a matter of debate. Certainly living with a person suffering from PTSD is stressful, and partners do show signs of emotional stress that increase in proportion to the severity of the trauma survivor's symptoms. And certain events in the relationships, such as violence or suicide attempts or threats, can be traumatic to the partner. But some research suggests that, apart from such direct trauma, the symptoms experienced by partners and their effects on marital satisfaction are accounted for primarily by caregiver burden.

Sexual Intimacy

As discussed in Chapter 9, sexual abuse and assault can affect physical intimacy in specific ways. Survivors of sexual trauma may feel anxiety about sex in general, during particular sexual activities, or when being touched in certain ways. They also may be prone to dissociation during sexual activity. The negative associations with physical intimacy and sexual arousal may cause some survivors of sexual assault and abuse to lose interest in sexual activity completely. Problems with sexual performance also can occur. Men who have experienced sexual abuse or assault sometimes have difficulty achieving erection, and women have trouble with arousal and achieving orgasm. Anxiety and shame related to sex may underlie these problems. If your partner is a survivor of sexual trauma, you might have noticed these difficulties, as well as problems with trust and intimacy in general. Also, some survivors of sexual abuse or assault experience "hypersexuality," or elevated desire for sex, which can alternate with periods of anxiety and inhibition or complete dissociation during sexual activity.

Difficulties with sex are not, however, limited to survivors of sexual trauma. Survivors of other types of trauma also might experience sexual problems, though primarily in association with PTSD.

One reason for this may be that sexual intimacy is so closely tied to intimacy in general. When PTSD affects the emotional connection between partners, they may become physically disconnected as well. In some cases, sexual relations may continue, but the partner may seem distant, absent, or, as Meagan experienced with Charlie, vacant or "robotic" during the experience. General emotional numbing might contribute to Charlie being numb during sex. PTSD can affect sexual desire, arousal, pleasure, and performance directly, as it can be difficult to fully relax and focus on the intimate contact. Problems with sexual performance, however, usually occur in combination with low libido. In some instances, unpleasant intrusive images might occur during intimacy, which can interfere with sexual performance and dampen interest in future sexual relations. Sexual problems also seem to coincide with high levels of anger. Finally, if your partner suffers from depression, this also can reduce interest in sex, along with interest in other pleasurable activities. Unfortunately, as discussed in Chapter 4, antidepressant medications prescribed for depression, PTSD, or related problems often have sexual side effects that can exacerbate these problems.

Sexuality is complex and influenced by many aspects of PTSD. Treatment for PTSD might result in improved sexual function, but if it does not, treatment methods designed specifically to address these problems can be of help. Raising the issue with a couple therapist, individual therapist, or physician is a good place to start if you are dissatisfied with your intimate relationship.

Conflict, Anger, and Violence

As discussed earlier, the elevated tendency to experience and express anger is one of the hyperarousal symptoms of PTSD. Some trauma survivors just feel irritable and angry without knowing why. Their anger may simply be the result of prolonged hyperarousal. Other survivors have specific sources of anger, many of which are justifiable. For example, Jim was angry because he knew that the factory fire was caused by negligence in the maintenance of machinery. Jim had previously reported the malfunctioning hardware to his supervisor, but the company had delayed the repairs. In addition, Jim was angry at the workers' compensation insurance company, which had been slow to pay for his surgeries and denied his claims for treatment of PTSD. Whenever he used his arm, he experienced pain to some degree, and he was reminded of his anger. So when Connie asked him to help with something as simple as setting the table for dinner, he hesitated. It wasn't that the pain was intolerable, but rather that he was afraid to trigger his anger. The trouble was, when he didn't do what Connie asked, she became angry with him. Then he felt guilty, so he withdrew to watch TV by himself. At least that way he didn't have to be reminded of the problems or that he was a burden to his wife.

For some trauma survivors, anger may be expressed as aggressive or violent behavior toward partners and family or toward others outside of the family. As discussed in Chapter 10, survivors of military trauma may be particularly prone to express anger through aggressive and violent behavior. More than half of American military veterans of the conflicts in Iraq and Afghanistan who have significant post-traumatic symptoms engage in some form of aggressive behavior. This is likely because military training and experience promote aggressive and violent behavior. Military trauma survivors are at elevated risk for engaging in violence toward their intimate partners. Surveys of U.S. military veterans estimate that one-third of veterans with PTSD have engaged in violence toward an intimate partner in the previous year—almost three times the rate for the general population. Approximately 90% engaged in some form of psychological aggression toward their partners. Veterans who abuse alcohol or drugs are more prone to both verbal and physical aggression (Taft et al., 2009).

Hyperarousal, depression, marital problems, and drug and alcohol abuse all seem to contribute to risk for physical violence. Veterans who engage in violence toward their partners may experience their hyperarousal as being out of their control. Psychologist Claude Chemtob has suggested that trauma survivors with PTSD may be prone to aggression because arousal puts them into "survival mode." Once in survival mode the trauma survivor will judge interactions with a partner to be potentially threatening. In this state, the trauma survivor with PTSD may be prone to misperceiving his partner's behavior as a threat to his safety, to which he might respond with violence to protect himself.

Trauma survivors who suffer from strong avoidance and emotional numbing symptoms of PTSD may be at higher risk for abusing their partners. It seems that these survivors have difficulty experiencing and expressing emotions to their partners, which reduces intimacy in their relationships. A partner's efforts to engage the trauma survivor may be perceived as irritating or insulting and can trigger aggression. The partner responds by distancing further from the survivor, which exacerbates the emotional disconnection. These survivors may benefit from treatment that helps them control aggressive impulses and increase emotional intimacy in their relationships.

If your loved one is prone to outbursts, then anger, hostility, and violence might be a part of your daily life. As we discussed in Chapter 1, you may feel inhibited about communicating feelings due to the trauma survivor's heightened sensitivity to anger. You may feel like you are "walking on eggshells" in an effort to avoid verbal or physical outbursts from the survivor. You might be living in fear due to having been the victim of her attacks or threats of violence or from witnessing your loved one engage in violent acts toward others. If your loved one is engaged in this pattern of violence, you may notice that you withdraw from him during these periods and that the rejection begets more anger and violence. You may feel that your family is stuck in a pattern of anger and violence that you cannot escape. You may consider the survivor the source of the problems in your family, and you may feel angry about the impact of his traumatic experiences on your lives. These factors can put your relationship at risk for separation or divorce. Also, your loved one may be at risk for suicide, discussed further below. In some instances the survivor may threaten suicide if you leave. And if he should engage in criminal assault, legal troubles might ensue. Often the survivor is aware that her aggressive and threatening behavior is out of control and a signal of deeper problems. She may nonetheless be reluctant to seek treatment. A trauma survivor who engages in aggressive or violent acts toward her partner, children, or others outside the family is in dire need of professional help.

A relationship that involves violence is complicated and presents a dilemma for you. You may feel love, compassion, commitment, and obligation toward your partner, and you may be concerned about the well-being of your children. Emotional bonds and moral obligations, combined with practical and financial constraints, can make leaving difficult, even when you're aware of clear dangers. But you should not try to persevere in such a situation on your own. If your loved one is unable or unwilling to seek professional help alone or with you, you should seek help for yourself. If your loved one has been violent toward you, domestic violence "hotlines" can be an important source of help. These agencies are typically staffed by volunteers from the community who are trained in the practical and legal aspects of managing situations involving family violence. You also may find professional counseling helpful in deciding whether to continue living with a partner who has been prone to violence.

Suicidal Thoughts, Threats, and Behaviors

Suicidal thoughts, threats, and behaviors are among the most alarming consequences of trauma exposure. Both PTSD and depression are associated with elevated risk for suicide. Persons suffering these aftereffects of trauma commonly contemplate suicide at some point. They also are more likely to attempt suicide compared to trauma survivors without such mental health diagnoses. Also, some survivors may engage in deliberate self-harm, such as cutting, burning, or scratching themselves without intending to end their lives. Often suicidal thoughts reflect the survivor's sense that he is a burden to others or that he "doesn't belong" or fit in with society. Feelings of shame and hopelessness often underlie suicidal impulses. Emotional disconnection within the survivor's primary intimate relationship can magnify the overall sense of "not belonging." Some trauma survivors use suicidal threats or gestures, such as cutting themselves, to communicate their distress to others. If your partner engages in this kind of behavior you might react strongly with fear, anger, sadness, and frustration.

As we stated earlier, if your traumatized partner has expressed suicidal urges, it is important to take them seriously. Most people who commit suicide have spoken to someone about their intent prior to doing so. Trauma survivors may be more likely to attempt suicide if they have access to a means of harming themselves, and the more lethal the method, the more likely the attempt will be successful. Use of alcohol and drugs also increases the likelihood of impulsive suicide attempts. If your partner has access to weapons, abuses alcohol or drugs, and has made verbal threats to harm himself, he may be at increased risk for suicide. Express your concern to him in a caring and nonjudgmental way. Let him know that his struggles are understandable. Encourage him to get professional help and go with him to the appointment. It is important to respond in a calm, supportive, and validating manner even if you are unsure of the seriousness of the threat.

Amanda had been growing more and more concerned about

Paul's gradual withdrawal from her, but she became alarmed when he mentioned killing himself one day while struggling with a repair in their apartment. After an hour under the kitchen sink, Paul came out, slammed his wrench on the ground, and mumbled, "Geez, why don't I just kill myself now?" Amanda had not thought Paul was particularly hopeless, but he did seem to be emotionally shut down, and she knew he had a pistol and a rifle and knew how to use them from his days in the military. Later, after he had put away his tools for the day, she asked him timidly whether he had been serious when he talked about killing himself. Paul first looked surprised, then scared, and then angry, and he told her that he was just joking and she shouldn't take him so seriously or listen to every single word he said. Paul got quiet, and just when Amanda thought she had driven him further away, he suddenly told her that he had thought a lot about killing himself, by using his pistol. Amanda tried to remain calm and supportive, but after a few moments she started to cry and told him that she was worried. Paul held her and said he didn't want to worry her, and he agreed to go see a therapist with her at the local VA that week. Amanda also asked him to leave his weapons with his father, and even though he grumbled about being in danger, he eventually agreed to do so.

Paul and Amanda were able to talk productively about Paul's feelings because they had a strong emotional connection. Not all conversations about suicidal thoughts will be as constructive. If you try to encourage your partner to seek help and she refuses, you may feel frustrated and frightened. Keep in mind that you can always call the police if you fear that your partner is in imminent danger and you can keep encouraging her to talk to a mental health professional. But if she won't do that, we encourage you to talk to a professional yourself for advice and support.

How Trauma Affects Children

Inasmuch as your partner's stress level affects you, it also may affect others living in the household. If you have children, you likely are concerned about how changes in your partner may be affecting them. A survivor's posttraumatic stress can affect family functioning in several ways.

When Your Partner Was the Only Family Member to Experience the Trauma

First, the emotional numbing and avoidance symptoms of PTSD may cause the parent to withdraw from the child. Fewer interactions with the child can interfere with developing a meaningful parent–child relationship and also can rob the child of valuable guidance and support. The child herself may seek less guidance and support if she senses that the parent is emotionally fragile because the parent avoids discussing the trauma or confronting reminders of it. Silence about the trauma can end up being a kind of "elephant in the room" that confuses and frightens the child as well.

Second, ambiguous loss may affect the child. She may not understand exactly why things have changed, but the child may notice her parents behaving differently and not fulfilling the same roles as before the trauma. Or, if the trauma occurred before the child was born, she might feel bereft when the parent with PTSD doesn't play as significant a role in her life as the other parent and isn't there for her in the same ways.

When children are confused about changes in the family, they may take responsibility for things they don't understand. For example, Paul's daughter, Sophie, who was in second grade when he left for Iraq, was excited when he came home 13 months later. She looked forward to doing things with him and fantasized about the fun they would have together. But 6 months after Dad's return, Sophie didn't understand why her father spent most of his time in his shop and hardly talked to her when he was around. She thought she had done something wrong and started thinking she was a "bad girl." Amanda noticed that Sophie seemed down, and her teachers said she wasn't paying attention in class and her grades were dropping. Amanda had no idea what was going through Sophie's head until she sat down with Sophie and talked about how Sophie felt about her father.

Children also may be affected by frequent exposure to the parent's reexperiencing and arousal symptoms. Some children may even mimic these behaviors. Also, if the parent discloses too much detail about the trauma, the child can become overwhelmed and frightened. This may be particularly true for younger children, because they don't understand many aspects of the trauma, such as those pertaining to sexuality and death. These children may develop symptoms of anxiety, fear, avoidance, even nightmares about what they imagine has happened to the parent or could happen to them or their family.

When Your Child Has Experienced Trauma Too

Many traumatic events, such as disasters and family violence, can be experienced directly by children along with their parents. Children also can be traumatized if the parent with PTSD engages in verbal or physical violence. Children are similarly susceptible to the effects of trauma and also can develop PTSD, although they may display their anxiety differently than adults. Some children may show their anxiety by saying that they feel sick and want to stay home from school and by withdrawing from playing with other children. Other children "act out" when they're feeling distress. Such children tend to get into fights with other kids and may be disobedient at home or school. Children who "internalize" their distress and those who "externalize" may both have trouble focusing on schoolwork, and their grades may drop.

When Your Partner's PTSD Affects You

The child of a trauma survivor with PTSD may be affected indirectly by how the PTSD affects you, the partner of the trauma survivor. If you are feeling the effects of caregiver burden, the added responsibility for your partner and the home may detract from the time and energy that you have to devote to your child. You may be feeling emotionally drained and at times lose your patience and be "snappy" with your child, or simply be emotionally unavailable to her. She may react by "being difficult." Your child may even feel that she must compete with your partner for your attention, which can create resentment.

In addition, as discussed above, you may be struggling to communicate your needs and resolve conflicts within the family. This can be more challenging when your partner with PTSD either explodes with anger or disengages entirely from you and your kids. You and your partner may disagree on parenting styles. Some parents with PTSD can become overcontrolling of their children's behavior, often because they have exaggerated concerns for their safety. Larissa had never allowed anyone to take care of their daughters besides her and Carlos. When they were teenagers, she made them tell her their whereabouts at all times, and this often caused fights with the girls, and with Carlos, who thought she was being overprotective.

What You Can Do to Repair Frayed Bonds

Everything we've recommended so far in this book, such as enhancing your understanding of what your loved one is going through, figuring out how you want to help, standing up for your own rights, and helping the survivor seek professional care if needed, will contribute to strengthening a relationship compromised by trauma. But there are resources designed specifically to help you two stick it out together, especially if you feel like the survivor you love is getting better but your relationship is still in danger.

Taking Care of Yourself

As noted above, the research shows that your overall distress and your dissatisfaction with your marriage are directly related to your sense of being burdened by caring for your traumatized partner. This points to the critical importance of reducing that sense of burden by taking care of yourself. Most partners of trauma survivors feel that they lack time for themselves, that they are too busy and exhausted, and that they are missing out on opportunities for enjoying themselves or pursuing their own goals in life. In earlier chapters we discussed skills for taking care of yourself, setting limits, and communicating assertively. These are critical tools for reducing your burden, which ultimately can reduce your stress, improve your marriage, and increase the likelihood that your partner will benefit from PTSD treatment.

As we discussed in Chapter 2, after a traumatic event, the survivor begins a pattern of coping that seems to help him get through the day. Avoiding reminders just seems to make sense and may even seem helpful in the short term. But in the long term, avoidance prevents adaptation, resolution, and healing from the events. Similarly, partners of trauma survivors do their best to manage all the upheaval in their lives. Like the trauma survivor's avoidant coping strategies, however, your ways of coping may jeopardize your long-term well-being as a couple.

You may tend to believe that your needs are less important than the survivor's, but ultimately, by not attending to your own needs, you hinder your partner's healing from his trauma and your own long-term well-being. For example, Amanda felt that she didn't deserve to take time for herself because she didn't suffer the awful events that her husband, Paul, had in Iraq. As a result, she gave up her weekly yoga class and no longer got together with her friends on Friday nights. Wanda took a second job in a retail store two nights a week and on weekends to make up for the lost income since Nadim had stopped working after the mugging. She felt exhausted all the time and often wished Nadim would pitch in, but then reminded herself that she wasn't the one who was mugged, so how could she understand how he felt? Wallace turned down an opportunity to take classes that would advance his career. He felt cheated out of the chance to improve his job situation, but he told himself that his goals weren't as important as Maria's needs.

It is critical that you set limits and boundaries with your partner—be sure to keep time for yourself, and don't bow to pressure to give up all of your personal, family, or professional activities and goals. In fact, consider taking up new activities that might contribute to your overall sense of personal fulfillment. If necessary, seek professional assistance for negotiating how to get your needs met in the context of your relationship with the trauma survivor. Consider joining a support group, either live or online, to help you get support to manage the burden you feel in caring for your partner. Your stress reduction is critical to your well-being and to the trauma survivor's recovery.

Taking Care of Your Relationship

Once you have made sure to attend to your own well-being, it is time to focus on the relationship. You can help your loved one with the decision to begin therapy, support her as she works through the healing process, or participate in couple therapy with your loved one.

Getting the Ball Rolling

The quality of intimate relationships has been shown to be important to successful PTSD treatment. When you have a better understanding of the symptoms with which your partner struggles, she may become more willing to share her feelings with you. This can help you feel closer to her and be more supportive of her in all phases of her recovery. Sometimes it may seem like your efforts to improve your relationship are futile—the more you try to engage your partner, the more she withdraws. Wallace felt like the harder he tried to be there for Maria, the more she backed away from him. Whenever he tried to talk with her about how things were going in their lives together, somehow they always ended up in a screaming match. Wallace decided to commit to working on improving their communication skills. He started with some of the basic strategies covered in Chapter 8. He discovered that when he started to share with Maria that he missed how they used to do things together, she began to let him in more on why she avoided doing some of those things. He started to realize that even small improvements in their communication could have a positive effect on their emotional connection. This was encouraging. Later, when he noticed that there was a group for families at the VA, he suggested they go together.

Conjoint CBT

Efforts are under way to develop treatment approaches to help couples in distress due to trauma. Psychologist Candace Monson has spearheaded efforts to develop a form of conjoint CBT specific to PTSD. Educating both partners about the effects of trauma exposure is a central aspect of these interventions. When the partner understands how emotional numbing and difficulties with intimacy are part of the overall reaction to trauma, he may be less inclined to react negatively to the trauma survivor's emotional withdrawal. By reading this book, you are well on your way to understanding your partner's reactions so that you can react more productively to your partner. Conjoint CBT also aims to improve emotional intimacy in two ways. First, it targets emotional numbing directly, because this is a core symptom that is so damaging to relationships. The trauma survivor is taught to label and express her feelings in the context of the marital relationship. Second, it teaches communication skills so that couples can deepen their intimacy by sharing emotions and expressing their needs to each other.

Conjoint CBT targets PTSD symptoms directly through the behavioral and cognitive therapy strategies discussed in Chapter 4. The therapy focuses on decreasing behavioral and experiential avoidance, similar to exposure therapy, and challenging thoughts and beliefs that influence PTSD and the relationship. Conjoint CBT is very new and still being tested with military veterans in the United States. As we noted earlier, much of the effect of trauma on veterans' relationships appears to be due to PTSD, not the type of trauma they experienced. So it is likely that conjoint CBT will be equally helpful for other types of trauma survivors.

Supporting PTSD Treatment

Although conjoint CBT is a promising approach, it is not yet widely available. It's important to realize, however, that PTSD underlies much of the distress experienced by both the trauma survivor and her partner. Therefore, resolving symptoms of PTSD in the trauma survivor is the top priority, as it has the potential to alleviate much of the strain on your relationship. Like Wallace, you can improve the quality of your relationship by being involved in your partner's treatment, whether by attending a family education or support group with her, joining in in an individual therapy session, or going together for couple therapy. Adding couple therapy to individual therapy for PTSD might achieve the same goal as conjoint therapy.

Couple Therapy

If your relationship is in jeopardy, it may be wise to begin couple therapy while the trauma survivor is working through individual therapy for PTSD. A good couple therapist can help you and your partner improve communication and conflict resolution skills, enhance sources of mutual pleasure, and restore emotional and physical intimacy. Reducing the strain of marital discord can go a long way in supporting the trauma survivor's efforts to resolve PTSD. If there has been violence in your intimate relationship, couple counseling may be particularly important. Although violence is a frequent reason that couples seek help, it is infrequently disclosed to the couple therapist. So if you have concerns about violence, be sure to disclose them in couple therapy so that the therapist can provide help for this serious problem. Talking about your partner's difficulties dealing with anger can be one way to open the door to discussing violence.

Anger Management Skills

Anger is a significant component of PTSD for many trauma survivors. As we have noted, its expression through aggressive behavior is a particular problem for survivors of military trauma. PTSD treatment can resolve anger problems for many trauma survivors, but not all will experience improvements in this area. For reasons not well understood, hyperarousal symptoms of PTSD often can persist even when the reexperiencing and avoidance symptoms have resolved. If your partner continues to show signs of aggression despite resolution of other aspects of his PTSD, then additional skills could be helpful. If aggression is a key impetus for seeking therapy, then treatment that teaches skills for managing anger and aggressive impulses might be helpful, particularly if the aggression persists after resolution of PTSD.

Anger management skills may be available in individual, group, or couple treatment formats and can include a wide variety of interventions. Typically, learning about the purpose of anger and how it is distinct from aggressive behavior serves as a foundation for other skills aimed at reducing arousal, correcting misattributions of others' behavior, communicating feelings and needs to others, negotiating conflicts, and solving problems. These types of skills have been shown to help reduce the intrusion of anger into daily life and reduce aggressive behavior. Many such programs aimed at preventing violent behavior are available in the community and at VA and military hospitals. Look for programs that focus on teaching specific skills for managing anger, rather than support groups or therapy groups that talk about what is beneath the anger.

Finally, you also should consider whether your partner's anger and irritability might be related to poor sleep. Like anger, sleep problems also can persist after resolution of PTSD, and in some cases the two may be related. If your partner is sleeping poorly despite resolution of nightmares, then cognitive-behavioral therapy for insomnia (see Chapter 4) might help.

Taking Care of Your Family

Increasingly, VA and military hospitals are offering family support programs, which can be a rich source for learning information and skills that can help you manage family issues. If these kinds of programs are available to you, keep them in mind as an invaluable resource. Family therapy, parenting classes, and support groups available from clinicians in the community also can be helpful, even if they are not focused specifically on families coping with PTSD. Trauma survivors suffering from PTSD might, however, be defensive about the possibility that their own problems might be having a negative effect on their children. This may make your partner reluctant to seek help as a family, even when such support services are available to you. You also might find that the burdens on you as a caregiver and provider of financial support would make it very difficult for you to attend family programs. If this is your situation, there are also numerous books and Internet resources to guide you in managing family problems. Some focus on addressing child behavior problems, improving communication, and teaching your children to communicate their emotions (see the Resources at the back of the book). Also keep in mind that encouraging your partner to get professional help is a priority because trauma survivors who get treatment for their PTSD are likely to show improvement in their family relationships. Working on improving your relationship also is key—reducing conflict in your relationship will help you provide the sense of safety and consistency that children need.

If you think your child could be suffering from PTSD, it's wise to seek professional counseling for her. There are adaptations of CBT specifically for children that are as effective as those for adults. If her anxiety symptoms are due to violence in the home, it's important to seek help for your child and yourself by establishing a safe home environment. Domestic violence agencies can provide the practical and legal support, and professional counseling can provide the emotional support and help with decision making, to establish safety for you and your child.

One way that PTSD affects children is by changing how family members communicate with one another. Studies of veterans with PTSD show that their families' communication and problem solving are not as good as those of families without PTSD. If your partner with PTSD tends to alternate between angry outbursts and withdrawal, it may be up to you to establish clear and direct communication with your children. You want to be sure that family rules and expectations are communicated clearly and respectfully. Also, it's important that you help your children learn to be aware of, and know how to talk about, their own feelings about daily issues as well as about PTSD. Make your relationship with your children a safe haven for them where they can talk about how they feel and get your help, support, and guidance in solving problems. Also, don't condone silence about the trauma, as children are likely to fill the void with their own ideas, which can lead to them feeling unnecessarily guilty, ashamed, or angry. But when you talk with children about your partner's trauma, be aware of what might be appropriate to share given their age and developmental stage and use age-appropriate language.

Focusing on your partner's needs can lead to changes in parenting styles and children's routines. Routines are important for children, helping them develop a sense of safety and predictability in the world. When their routines are disrupted, they may feel stressed and start behaving differently or complaining of feeling sick rather than talking about how they feel. You can help your children by maintaining your normal family routines and expectations. Keep in mind that there is very limited research into the effects of parental trauma on children, so it's not clear that all children are at risk for problems. Some children can be affected when the traumatized parent has PTSD, but not all children in the same family are affected in the same way. You can help to mitigate the effects of your partner's PTSD on your children by providing the consistency, clear boundaries, open communication, and support that children need.

Building Emotional Connection

If there is one thing we know about relationships, it's that emotional connections sustain them. Being in a relationship with a trauma survivor can be challenging and stressful in so many ways. You may feel exhausted by the daily burdens of caring for your partner and family and just keeping things together. You may be struggling to keep the peace in a household where chaos seems to reign. Or you may be feeling sad, lonely, and isolated living with a partner who shuts out the world. When things seem out of control, you might get caught up in blaming your partner for so many of the problems in your lives together.

Amid the emotional turmoil and frustration it's easy to lose sight of what brought you together. While working to solve the problems in your lives, it also is critical that you work on nurturing your emotional connection to each other. Express your mutual appreciation and affection on a daily basis and set aside time to connect with each other weekly. Be willing to overlook each other's flaws and look into each other's eyes. Cherish each other's assets. Relationships that thrive are not without conflicts, but they do show a higher proportion of praise, expressions of appreciation, and affection relative to the number of negative interactions. Be open to your partner's ideas and willing to grow from your experiences together. Most important, respond to each other's emotional needs. For your relationship to survive and flourish, you must not only work to resolve conflicts but also deliberately nurture your sense of mutual respect, caring, and appreciation for what each of you brings to your life together.

TWELVE

Recovery and Beyond

The change in Marcus was amazing. He wasn't scared of the world anymore, and he had gotten back into his old hobbies like woodworking and building model planes and had even picked up some new ones. He was sleeping through the night, and the memories no longer bothered him. It was clear that his deployment still affected him; he still periodically broke down in tears when he was reminded of the men he had served with in Iraq who had not come back alive. And he still got irritated really easily when he heard people complaining about how "hard" life is. But treatment had made a major difference. The biggest change was the way he had embraced life. He was constantly trying new things and going places he had never been, and instead of telling Marion how dangerous the world was, he encouraged her to get out and experience things. She asked him once what had changed. He smiled and told her that sometime during his therapy it dawned on him what a precious thing life is. He still believed that it could be taken at any time, but now he was focused on doing all he could while he still had the chance. "Every day is a gift," he said with a smile. "The guys I lost, they don't get that gift. How can I turn it down?"

Juan had hoped that his life with Estelle might eventually return to the way it had been, but he had never imagined things could actually be better. Estelle was pretty much her old self—more cautious, to be sure, but running and volunteering at the Humane Society again and back to spending time with her friends. It was their rela-

tionship that had changed. One evening as they drove home from a session with her therapist, Estelle turned to him and said she'd never forget how he had been there for her and how he'd been willing to do anything for her. She knew now that she could count on him for anything. After that, they both seemed not to get caught up in the petty little things they had always argued about. The depth of their mutual trust and connection was evident in their daily lives, and he felt richer for it. They both seemed to realize that, compared to dealing with a rape, being late on a bill or finding out the car needed brakes was nothing to worry about. It was almost like they had been tested in fire and come out stronger.

Tom was just about back to normal. He still drove really slowly, and Joe sometimes couldn't believe how long he spent sitting at stop signs while he made sure no one was coming. But Tom was back out there, and that was the most important thing. At one point the topic of the crash came up, and Joe told Tom how glad he was that all of that was behind them. Tom only shrugged and said, "That whole episode taught me one thing—that if I work, I can get over just about anything." Joe was surprised—after all, it was clear that Tom still had some trouble driving. How could he see it as a beneficial event if it still bothered him?

Life can be overwhelming in the aftermath of trauma. We hope that understanding the effects of trauma has helped you support your loved one more effectively as well as attend to your own needs. If you've discovered that this book isn't enough to help you both cope, we hope our guidance has helped you get the professional help you need. Most of all, we hope this book has trained your eye on the very real possibility of recovery—and even growth.

Recovery Is Possible

Trauma, by its nature, changes people in profound and often permanent ways. But PTSD is not something a survivor must learn to live with. Rather, it consists of normal reactions to danger, the intensity of which can be reduced when the survivor relearns a sense of safety in her present life. By facing fears and reexamining the meaning of the traumatic event, through therapy if necessary, your loved one can resolve sources of distress and resume a balanced and emotionally healthy life. Therapy also can reduce worry, brighten mood, normalize eating, and allow sound and restorative sleep.

As we've noted, the road to recovery is often bumpy, especially because many survivors either are reluctant to seek help or have trouble staying with treatment. Yet with treatment, the traumatic event that once was devastating can become one of many tales in life's story, which, though still poignant, no longer need be agonizing. Research has consistently shown that those who complete treatment fare better than those who drop out, and treatment benefits not only the survivor but also loved ones, whose lives will be less disrupted by the fallout of PTSD.

With your help, we hope your loved one will recover much of the quality of life that was lost as a result of the trauma. In her struggle to cope with the trauma, your loved one also might experience positive transformations in her outlook on life and overall well-being. Perhaps surprisingly, such positive changes have long been recognized among trauma researchers. And you might share in them, benefiting directly and also experiencing a trickle-down of positive effects from the survivor's changes. The rest of this chapter describes specific strategies for nurturing positive growth after trauma that can be used to benefit you both.

Before we embark on this discussion, please understand that, while we feel it's important to present the more optimistic side of the trauma story, many trauma survivors do not experience growth, and there's no evidence that positive changes are essential for recovery. Conversely, recovery is not a prerequisite for positive change—you might be surprised to learn that positive changes can occur even when some degree of distress persists. Regardless, it is important to realize that although we want to shine a light on the *possibility* of positive change, this kind of change need not be the goal. If your loved one does not show the kinds of positive reactions discussed here, he may be no worse for it.

Positive Change Also Can Happen

The notion of positive changes resulting from trauma may seem counterintuitive. So far in this book we've focused on the negative ways that trauma can affect both you and your loved one. And from your own experience you've probably thought that the traumatic event has caused only trouble in your lives. But the effects of trauma are not necessarily *all* negative. As you support your loved one in the process of recovering from trauma, you may find that you both grow from the experience and become stronger. You may watch as your loved one emerges from trauma a more resourceful and confident person. Over time you may become aware that you yourself don't worry as much about certain things anymore. After having supported your loved one through very difficult times, you may be less likely to "sweat the small stuff."

Trauma researchers have noticed that some people who experience trauma learn and grow from the event in positive ways. They emerge from their ordeals stronger and more confident, with a richer appreciation of life and deeper, more satisfying relationships. Researchers Lawrence Calhoun and Richard Tedeschi (2006) have been studying positive transformation in the aftermath of trauma for over 20 years. They've observed that trauma can lead to positive changes in personal strength, relationships with others, spirituality, the ability to see new and alternate possibilities in life, and greater appreciation of life.

Learning Strength

Many survivors struggle so much with the aftereffects of trauma, or try so hard to avoid thinking about the event, that they never really consider that they survived something very difficult. Similarly, the survivor as well as her loved ones may not see how much she accomplished in coping with the problems caused by the trauma. Recognizing the magnitude of what was overcome can help survivors and their loved ones come fully to realize their strength.

In the course of working through the memories of the trauma, the survivor may realize that she lived through something very dangerous, and this can increase her belief that she can handle difficult situations. Most traumatic events involve real or threatened harm, and the survivor may have had to struggle to stay alive or help others. When the survivor recognizes that she was strong enough to emerge from the trauma alive, this can bolster her confidence in her own strength. Sarah was surprised when the police called her 2 weeks after her assault to inform her that they had apprehended her attacker. She was able to pick him out of a lineup, and the officers told her he would probably go to jail. A week before the trial, he arrived at her doorstep with a gun, but when she saw him outside she called the police and fled out the back door. Sarah felt scared but also felt triumphant when he was caught—she had survived. She felt brave when she faced him in court, and she stared him right in the face. You tried, she thought, but you couldn't stop me. You're going to jail. After the trial was over, Sarah found herself feeling more confident in many situations at work and in her social life. She had survived a horrible ordeal. Why should she worry about a project at work or meeting someone new?

This increased sense of strength can sometimes develop as the survivor processes her experiences in therapy. For several years after serving as a medic in Afghanistan, Maria struggled with guilt about one mass-casualty event in which she had to decide which wounded soldiers received treatment and which were beyond saving. It was a horrible experience, and she couldn't help feeling that she should have done more to save all of them. Early in treatment, Maria's therapist recognized that her belief that she should have saved more was a major source of guilt and distress. After several sessions of cognitive therapy, Maria concluded that there was no way she could have helped all of the wounded. She also realized that because of her quick and decisive action, everyone who had a chance to live was saved. She then started thinking about all the other times she had saved wounded soldiers, and she began to feel proud of herself. She realized that she had accomplished a lot under very difficult circumstances. Instead of doubting herself, she began to believe that she was a smart, resourceful, and capable person.

Some trauma survivors also feel stronger as a result of facing their fears in therapy. After Estelle's first session of imaginal exposure focused on her memory of the assault, she felt shaky but good. She had done it—she had faced up to the thing she feared most, and she hadn't backed down. It had been scary, but she got through it, and what's more, her therapist had been right—she wasn't as anxious at the end of the exposure as she had been when it started. She learned that if she faced her fears, and did so with the support of the people around her, she could conquer them, and this was an empowering lesson. After she completed treatment, she decided she would face other fears that had limited her. She had always loved running, and she knew she was fast, but she had always shied away from entering races, because she just didn't feel confident. Since her therapy, she not only got back into running, but she decided to take it more seriously and train for a half-marathon.

Some survivors emerge from their experiences with more tenacity and persistence in the face of adversity. The survivor realizes that she's stronger than she thought and that she can trust that strength enough to stick with a difficult task longer and not give up easily. In an effort to be around people more as part of her therapy, Estelle started playing softball in Juan's recreational league. She was not very good, but she surprised Juan by continuing to play and working to improve herself as a player. At the end of the season Juan overheard another player compliment Estelle on how far she had come in one season. She smiled, thanking him, and said, "Well, I've faced a lot tougher stuff than a softball."

Your experiences in dealing with your loved one's trauma might also lead you to discover that you are stronger than you once thought. As you learn to manage your own reactions to changes in your loved one, improve your self-care, and offer support to the survivor in your life, you may emerge with increased confidence in your capabilities. Two years after Mark returned from Afghanistan, he had readjusted to the civilian world, was sleeping through the night, and was working full-time. He still doted on the boys, but he was much more of a disciplinarian than he had been. One night, as she watched Mark and the boys playing in the yard after a barbecue, Eva smiled to herself. She had kept her family together, taken care of herself and her boys, and helped her husband get his life back on track. She felt a quiet sort of confidence. She knew that life would have other challenges for her, but she also felt confident that she could handle whatever life dished out to her.

New Possibilities

Another positive transformation that can happen for some trauma survivors and their loved ones is the ability to see new possibilities in life. This can mean taking on new hobbies or interests, shifting priorities in what matters and how you spend your time, or even changing career paths. As he simultaneously processed the trauma and adjusted to the civilian world, Marcus was able to balance his love for the military with his return to his job and family. Once he resolved his own judgments about his experiences, he no longer felt like he had to avoid questions about the war or his service. He felt comfortable wearing all of his Army T-shirts and hats and reconnected with several soldiers with whom he had deployed. In fact, it seemed to Jenny that Marcus had gone from avoiding to trying to inform people. At one of Marion's field hockey games, a friend of hers asked Marcus whether he had killed anyone. Marcus became serious and told the boy that questions like that weren't appropriate to ask someone who had been to war. Marcus said that killing was a very intense thing and not a conversation topic for discussion at a sports event. But he offered to tell the teenager about the Army if he ever wanted to know. When Jenny asked him why he had taken the time to explain all that, Marcus said he had been to war and many others had not—if he didn't at least try to explain what war is, how could civilians ever know? How could they make up their minds about the direction of the country or vote? Jenny had never thought that Marcus would come to see himself as a war veteran who could reach out to others.

Loved ones might find themselves undergoing a similar transformation. As they helped their son, Todd, through the treatment process, Ellie and Keith learned more and more about the VA and its services for veterans. They were incredibly relieved when Todd was able to manage his anxiety and anger better and started sleeping more. When he finally got a job and moved out, they almost didn't know what to do with themselves. Ellie was glad to get back to life as usual, but for Keith the idea of other veterans like Todd struggling on their own was too much to bear. So he started a website for younger veterans in his state who had not yet gone to the VA for help. He posted as much "inside information" as he could about Todd's experiences and what they had learned about VA benefits for which he was eligible. He started a message board on the site and was amazed as veterans started to share their own triumphs and concerns with each other. Keith took pride in his role as activist and realized that helping people was something he cared about and found rewarding.

Solidifying Relationships

In the same way that trauma can strengthen you and your loved one, it also can strengthen your relationship with each other. Relationships are more than just the sum of two individuals—they are entities unto themselves, which can be nurtured and grow or be ignored and allowed to decline. Sometimes the ordeal of coping with trauma and its effects can drive people apart. In other cases, when people are able to commit to each other and to the relationship, the process of change can increase levels of trust and caring.

In Chapter 1 we talked about the confusion, isolation, and loss of intimacy you may have experienced after the trauma. In Chapter 2, we discussed how trauma may have affected the survivor's ability to trust as well as his difficulty feeling an emotional connection with others. In Chapter 11 we looked at the effects of trauma on relationships and families. If you committed to staying with the survivor and helping him, then recovery from trauma can restore your sense of who he is. Jenny often had felt confused by the changes she saw in Marcus and had wondered whether he would ever be back to normal. But as he slowly engaged in treatment and opened up more and more to her about his struggles, she realized he was still the same man, still her husband, whom she had known for almost 20 years. He was just dealing with horrific events that she had never seen him deal with, and it was hard for him. And even as he recovered and she realized that some things would never go back to the way they were, she still felt connected with him. Some of his views had changed, and choices he made were different, but at his core he was still Marcus. As you watch your loved one recover and notice the changes that occur during the recovery process, keep in mind that he is still the same person. This can help you see these changes in the context of the person you have always known and been close to, which in turn can help you stay close to him as he recovers and grows as a person.

Without sufficient commitment to a relationship, a crisis can drive loved ones apart. As you face and work through obstacles together, you may find that you and your loved one grow *closer*. When both parties are committed to the relationship and to each other, crises can deepen and strengthen bonds between them. Diane and Roger definitely had their share of arguments while Roger got accustomed to his group at the VA and then started working on his anger and nightmares. But as Roger started to make positive changes in his life, he and Diane just seemed to get closer and closer, as if with each step they were reminded of how much they cared for each other. Although they had been married for almost 30 years, Roger and Diane felt closer to each other than they had when they were young. They each felt they had learned a lot about their partner and themselves through the recovery process. The improvement in their communication had deepened their understanding of each other's needs and perspectives. They came to appreciate how fortunate they were to have each other.

If you draw on your own sources of social support as you cope with the survivor's recovery process, you may find that your relationships with the people who support you also are strengthened. You may learn that people in your life really do care about you, and this may increase your level of trust in them. Throughout Marcus's recovery, Jenny continued to meet regularly with the other wives from his platoon. Even as Marcus improved, she continued to spend time with them, and as they endured their own difficulties she tried to be as supportive and helpful as she could. Over time those supportive relationships turned into friendships, and Jenny realized that she had new people in her life whom she could count on in times of crisis. She thought about how reluctant she had been to open up to the other women when Marcus was first deployed, and looking back, she was glad that she had taken the risk.

Recovery can not only restore but also enhance the trust that your loved one has in you. Juan had never doubted that he loved Estelle— not for a second. But after he committed to staying with her through her hardships, and after she trusted him enough to confide in him and involve him in her recovery, he felt closer to her than ever before. Estelle learned that she could trust Juan with her deepest fears and he would always be there to help. Juan learned how much he loved his wife, how much he was willing to do for her, and how good that felt to him. Tom had always known that his brother would be there for him, but as he dealt with the car crash and the problems that followed, he really understood how much he could trust his brother. A couple of times, Joe had given Tom feedback about how Tom was living his life, but he always seemed to have Tom's best interests in mind, and that meant a lot to Tom. He realized that he could always count on his brother to be there for him.

Making the commitment to support the trauma survivor in your life can draw you closer together, whether the trauma survivor is a spouse, child, sibling, or friend. Your support can serve as evidence of how much she means to you and how much you care.

Spiritual Deepening

Trauma inevitably brings up questions of why things happen, and for some these questions lead to a search for meaning. Sometimes the survivor and her loved one can find profound and positive answers to these deep questions within their spirituality. As Ike watched his daughter, Karen, struggle with bad memories about her deployment, he worried about her and wondered why she had to go through this. After all, she had volunteered to serve her country. Why should she suffer? Then Karen started going to the VA, and 6 months later she seemed like a different person. She met Ike for lunch one day and told him she had come to believe she was meant to help other vets who weren't fortunate enough to have parents like hers. Ike was touched. He concluded that in the end Karen's horrible experiences in the war had been put into her life to strengthen her and give her life purpose.

After he was attacked, Nadim went through a period when he lost his faith and stopped going to church or otherwise thinking about god. Wanda was worried, because he had always been a religious person. She didn't think it was her place to tell him what he should believe, so she didn't push him. Instead, she let him work things out on his own. At the very end of his therapy, Nadim confided in Wanda that he had resolved how god could have allowed the mugging to happen. He said that he used to read things in the Bible about bad things happening to good people, but he had never really understood it. Now he did, and he felt that much closer to god. He actually said that if the trauma had not happened he would not have understood what it meant to suffer and persevere in his faith. Wanda wasn't totally sure how he had come to that understanding, but she was glad that he had reconciled his experience with his beliefs and that he was back in church.

Appreciating Life

You may recall from Chapter 2 that some trauma survivors develop a sense of a foreshortened future or the belief that life can be cut short at any moment. For some survivors, this belief can lead to depression and lack of motivation. Other survivors can find meaning in that belief, and that meaning can serve as motivation for living a valued life. Years after his sister Kate witnessed a severe accident at work, Sean threw a party to celebrate his daughter Siobhan's 16th birthday. Kate, Siobhan's favorite aunt, gave her a huge hug and told her how glad she was that Siobhan had made it to 16. Sean felt a little uncomfortable and commented to Kate that she sounded a little morbid. Kate smiled and said, "No, I'm really happy for her. You can't take anything for granted. It's all a gift!" She then turned to Siobhan, hugged her again, and told her to appreciate every day she had and treat each moment as something special.

Are There Ways to Foster Positive Change?

Whether we can train people to be less vulnerable to the negative effects of trauma and more likely to experience positive changes has been a subject of interest to many psychologists. Donald Meichenbaum, the developer of stress inoculation training (introduced in Chapter 4), has distinguished between ways of thinking that keep one stuck in the past and those that help a person move forward (Meichenbaum, 2006). He notes that people who get stuck in the past focus on certain trains of thought, such as assigning blame, viewing themselves as victims (mentally defeated or permanently changed), trying to figure out how the event could have been prevented (rather than accepting what happened), brooding about and pining for the past, and blurring boundaries between the past and present (seeing ongoing threat and impending doom in the present). Until her therapy, Estelle kept thinking, "I should have known it wasn't safe." After the rape, Tess believed, "My reputation is ruined forever." When he first came back from Iraq, Paul was stuck thinking, "If only I hadn't fired when the commander said to." Freddie thought, "If only things could go back to the way they were before the accident." After the sexual assault, Hank was focused on the thought, "I've been betrayed; no one can be trusted."

Perhaps you've caught yourself thinking this way too. Jenny often thought, "I wish I had the old Marcus back." Maggie sometimes wished Tess had never gone to the party. Patricia often grumbled that "the company should pay for what they did to Freddie." Although you may not experience the stress in the same way as the trauma survivor, this way of thinking could keep you stuck along with the survivor in your life.

The table on the next page shows ways of thinking that can help foster positive change. Finding benefit for yourself or others, comparing yourself to others who might be worse off, looking to the future, and constructing meaning out of the experience all can help you grow and change in positive ways.

Psychologist Martin Seligman has focused on how we can enhance resilience against the negative effects of trauma. His program, which uses cognitive behavioral methods to enhance emotional resilience, is being taught throughout the U.S. Army to see whether building emotional resilience can prevent PTSD. The approach emphasizes teaching optimistic and constructive ways of thinking, assertive communication, problem solving, decision-making skills, and relaxation skills. These are some of the same tools and skills that we have introduced in this book, so there is a good chance that practicing these skills will help you be "inoculated" against the effects of stress, including the stress of coping with the trauma survivor in your life.

The American Psychological Association provides a useful guide called "The Road to Resilience" (www.apa.org/helpcenter/road-resilience.aspx) that offers guidance for nurturing emotional well-being in the face of life stress. It points to 10 things to focus on in your life that can help you be less vulnerable to the negative effects of stress and more likely to experience positive outcomes. These suggestions, explained in more detail on the website, may help both you and the trauma survivor. When communicating with the trauma survivor in your life, keep in mind that some people can be put off by the suggestion that they

Ten Ways to Build Resilience

1. Make connections.
2. Avoid seeing crises as insurmountable problems.
3. Accept that change is a part of living.
4. Move toward your goals.
5. Take decisive actions.
6. Look for opportunities for self-discovery.
7. Nurture a positive view of yourself.
8. Keep things in perspective.
9. Maintain a hopeful outlook.
10. Take care of yourself.

Kinds of Thinking and Behaviors That Lead Survivors toward "Growth"

Thinking pattern	Prototypic examples
Benefit seeking, finding, and reminding—SELF	"I am wiser (stronger) as a result of this experience." "I am better prepared for whatever comes along." "I am less afraid of change." "I never knew I could get along on my own." "I am better now at helping others."
Benefit seeking, finding, and reminding—OTHERS	"This brought us all together." "I learned I am my brother's keeper." "I learned not to immerse myself in other people's pain."
Engage in downward comparison	"I think about others and how it could have been worse." "I recognize that I need to accept help." "My view of what is important in life has changed."
Establish a future orientation	"My view of what is important in life has changed." "I see new possibilities and goals to work on." "I am now able to focus on the fact that it happened to me and not on how it happened."
Constructing meaning	"We survived and we have a chance to live, and we're choosing life." "I am no longer willing to be defined by my victimization." "I survived for a purpose. I accept that responsibility. I owe it to those who perished to tell their stories (honor their memory, share with others, prevent this from happening again)." "I moved from being a victim to becoming a survivor and even a thriver." "I can make a gift of my pain and loss to others." "I now know God."

Note. Adapted from Meichenbaum (2006). Copyright 2006 by Lawrence Erlbaum Associates. Adapted with permission from the Copyright Clearance Center.

should grow or change in positive ways from a negative experience—that they should see something positive amid all the horror. So avoid giving simple advice about staying positive, such as "You really ought to look on the bright side" or "You're being entirely too negative—you need to start thinking more positively about things." You may find it more effective to focus on modeling your own constructive thinking about the situation with statements such as "As bad as it was, it brought us together, and for that I am very grateful" or "What you went through was so horrible, it really made me realize what's important in life." By commenting on your own thoughts rather than the survivor's and simply sharing your alternative point of view, you avoid being overly critical of the survivor but still can increase his awareness of alternative perspectives. These kinds of disclosures have the added benefit of enhancing your mutual intimacy.

The utility of the skills that you and your loved one learn in the course of support and recovery is not limited to coping with trauma. These skills can be applied to many different situations in life. Aaron occasionally had to work long days, and sometimes the late-afternoon meetings on those days were stressful. Although his job didn't remind him of Afghanistan in any way, he was able to use the muscle relaxation he had learned in therapy to help him reduce his stress at work and get through the day in a better mood. Greg set aside a half-hour every evening to ride his exercise bike and do jumping jacks and push-ups to make sure he had enough energy and slept well while his girlfriend, Jeanette, was in treatment. He was ecstatic when Jeanette was able to take control of her life again, but Greg kept exercising. It made him feel healthier; why stop? When Nadim and Wanda were trying to decide whether to move out of their apartment to a building in a nicer part of town, Wanda pulled out a pro–con form. Nadim took one look at it, rolled his eyes, and said, "Oh, come on, I thought I was done with therapy!" They had a laugh and then used the form to look at all the reasons to move or to stay in their old place.

As you travel on the long road of recovery, it can be difficult to think you're doing anything right. We recommend setting small goals along the way and recognizing your accomplishments. Don't wait to congratulate yourself until your loved one is back at work, no longer bothered by bad memories, and sleeping through the night. Instead, pat yourself on the back as often as possible throughout the recovery process. When Estelle went to her first therapy session, Juan was thrilled. He told himself that it had taken a lot of effort but they had accomplished something, and that was a great start that they could build on. He knew they still had a long way to go, but something had changed, and that meant other things could too. Like Juan, you can build your sense of strength and your hope along the way as you support your loved one.

A Final Word: Trauma and the Fabric of Your Life

Throughout human history, many authors have written about our existence as a fabric or tapestry, with each person's experiences woven into the larger context of the rest of his life. Each part of the tapestry has its own specific characteristics or appearance, but all parts come together as one unified whole. The more we can see the whole tapestry and the course of our life, the easier it is to integrate subsequent experiences into our life story, and the less those experiences will affect us. As you reflect on how trauma has affected your loved one, and as you recover from the effects that your loved one's trauma has had on you, it can be useful to think of your own life this way.

Recovery, for you and the survivor, means weaving the trauma and all its effects into the fabric of life. Before the recovery process, the trauma stood alone, and it seemed like life as you knew it had stopped and something new and unfamiliar took its place. The trauma prevented you from moving forward and kept you stuck right where you were. As you and the survivor recover, you integrate the trauma and all its effects into your life. It becomes a part of your life experiences, woven into the fabric. It may have a different color and texture from the rest of the fabric, but it is part of it nonetheless.

The traumatic event happened, and it affected your loved one. It will always be a part of her life. As we've said again and again in this book, the more the survivor tries to push it away and struggles against it, the more it keeps her from moving on. When she lets go of the struggle and faces her fears, the effects of trauma may decrease and even disappear over time. Because the survivor is close to you, the trauma and its effects are part of your life, too. The harder you fight against that, the more you will stay stuck. If you commit to using the skills we have talked about in this book to support your loved one and take care of yourself, you too can process your experience of the trauma and integrate it into your life. It will be woven into the tapestry like any other experience you have had. When this happens, you and the survivor will be able to move forward and continue weaving the fabric of your lives.

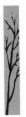

Resources

Organizations

Australia

Australian Psychological Society
www.psychology.org.au

Department of Veterans Affairs
www.dva.gov.au/
    The Veterans and Veterans Families Counselling Service provides 24-hour crisis telephone counselling services:

- VVCS: 1-800-011-046
- Lifeline: 13-11-14
- SANE Helpline: 1-800-18-SANE (7263)

National Brain Injury Foundation
www.nbif.org.au
    Dedicated to assisting those with acquired brain injury and their families.

16 Birdwood Street, Hughes, ACT
PO Box 5542, Hughes, ACT 2605
Phone: (02) 6282 2880 (Monday–Friday, 9:00 A.M.–5:00 P.M.)
Fax: (02) 6285-2649
E-mail: *manager@nbif.org.au*

Australian Centre for Posttraumatic Mental Health at the University of Melbourne
www.acpmh.unimelb.edu.au

Level 1, 340 Albert Street
East Melbourne, VIC 3002
Phone: (61) 3-9936-5100
Fax: (61) 3-9936-5199
Email: *acpmh-info@unimelb.edu.au*
For immediate assistance or support, call Lifeline on 13-11-14 for confidential 24-hour counseling and referrals.

Belize, Central America

Ministry of Health
www.health.gov.bz/www/index.php/units/mental-health
Provides integrated, comprehensive, accessible mental health services, focusing on promotion, prevention, early detection, treatment, and rehabilitation, and emphasizing community-based services and respect for the human rights of people with mental illness and their care providers.

Canada

Canadian Psychological Association
www.cpa.ca

Health Canada
www.hc-sc.gc.ca/index-eng.php
Information and resources for a variety of health care issues, including mental health.

The PTSD Association
www.ptsdassociation.com/index.php

Veterans Affairs Canada
www.veterans.gc.ca
Offers information and links to National Centre for Operational Stress Injuries (NCOSI), which cooperates with its partners to ensure the development, delivery, and coordination of clinical mental health services. The NCOSI also contributes to the advancement and dissemination of knowledge and practices regarding clinical services, particularly in the field of operational stress injuries.

New Zealand

Mental Health Foundation of New Zealand
www.mentalhealth.org.nz
   Provides information, evidence-based research, and best practice; facilitates understanding; and offers support.

E-mail: *info@mentalhealth.org.nz*
Phone: (09) 300-7030

Veterans and Veterans Families Counselling Service (VVCS)
Phone: 1-800-011-046

South Africa

Mental Health Information Centre of South Africa
www.sahealthinfo.org/mentalhealth/consumerinfo.htm
   Offers information about mental health as well as links to directories of service providers.

United Kingdom

Combat Stress
www.combatstress.org.uk
   Combat Stress is the United Kingdom's leading military charity, specializing in the care of veterans' mental health, including delivery of dedicated treatment and support to ex-service men and women with conditions such as PTSD, depression, and anxiety disorders. Services free of charge to veterans.

Tyrwhitt House, Oaklawn Road
Leatherhead, Surrey KT22 0BX
Phone: 01372-587000
E-mail: contactus@combatstress.org.uk

Counselling Directory
www.counselling-directory.org.uk
   Lists qualified/registered counselors and psychotherapists and offers numerous articles and sources of information about PTSD and the effects of trauma. Also some FAQs on how to choose a therapist and what counseling/psychotherapy means.

Reach Out
ie.reachout.com
   Inspires young people to help themselves through tough times and find ways to improve their own mental health and well-being by building skills and providing information, support, and referrals in ways that work for young people. Run by the Inspire Ireland Foundation (www.inspireireland.ie), whose mission is to help young people lead happier lives.

The Royal College of Psychiatrists
www.rcpsych.ac.uk/mentalhealthinfo/problems/ptsd/posttraumaticstressdisorder.
aspx

17 Belgrave Square
London SW1X 8PG
Phone: 020-7235-2351, ext. 6259

UK Trauma Group
www.ukpts.co.uk/site/trauma-services
   A managed clinical network and resource for advice and information for the general public and for health professionals about posttraumatic stress reactions.

United States

U.S. Military and Veterans

Afterdeployment.org
www.afterdeployment.org
   A mental wellness resource for service members, veterans, and military families.

American Veterans with Brain Injuries
www.avbi.org
   A peer chat room and forum for American service members and veterans, as well as for family members and caregivers. Both the forum and chat room are interactive and designed for participants to ask questions, get information, and share personal experiences with others.

Association of the United States Army
www.ausa.org
   AUSA's "Family Programs Directorate" is dedicated to providing Army families with information and resources to help them manage the challenges of military life and to addressing Army family concerns through legislative efforts and by being active on a number of Department of Defense and Department of the Army councils and working groups.

Brain Injury Association of America
www.biausa.org
   Devoted to creating a better future through brain injury prevention, research, education and advocacy, the BIAA offers extensive resources and links to related websites.

Phone: 1-800-444-6443

Brain Trauma Foundation (BTF)

www.braintrauma.org

Dedicated to improving the outcome of traumatic brain injury (TBI) patients worldwide by developing best practices guidelines, conducting clinical research, and educating medical professionals and consumers.

7 World Trade Center
34th Floor
250 Greenwich Street
New York, NY 10007
Phone: 212-772-0608

Brainline.org

www.brainline.org

A national multimedia project offering information and resources about preventing, treating, and living with TBI, funded by Defense and Veterans Brain Injury Center (DVBIC) and a service of WETA, the public TV and radio station in Washington, DC.

Courage to Care Campaign

www.usuhs.mil/psy/courage.html

Provides fact sheets relevant to military life developed by experts from the Uniformed Services University of the Health Sciences (USUHS).

Defense and Veterans Brain Injury Center

www.dvbic.org

Give an Hour

www.giveanhour.org

A nonprofit group providing free mental health services to U.S. military personnel and families affected by the current conflicts in Iraq and Afghanistan.

Military OneSource

www.militaryonesource.com

Service members, veterans, and families can call 24/7 to speak to a master's-level consultant.

Phone: in the United States, 1-800-342-9647; outside the United States, (country access code) 800-342-9647 (dial all 11 numbers)
International toll-free: 1-800-464-8107

My HealtheVet

www.myhealth.va.gov

My HealtheVet is the new Veterans Health Administration health portal created for veterans and their families, as well as for VA employees. It enables you to access health information, tools, and services anywhere in the world you can access the Internet.

The National Center for PTSD

www.ptsd.va.gov

Aims to help U.S. veterans and others through research, education, and training on trauma and PTSD; offers information about PTSD and links to assist you in locating VA facilities and mental health services in your area.

ReMIND

www.remind.org

The Bob Woodruff Foundation provides resources and support to injured service members, veterans, and their families, building a movement to empower communities nationwide to take action to successfully reintegrate our nation's injured heroes—especially those who have sustained the "hidden injuries of war"—back into their communities so they may thrive physically, psychologically, socially, and economically.

ReMIND
Bob Woodruff Foundation
PO Box 955
Bristow, VA 20136
E-mail: *info@ReMIND.org*

Sesame Street's Talk, Listen, Connect: Deployments, Homecomings, Changes

www.sesameworkshop.org/initiatives/emotion/tlc

A bilingual educational outreach initiative designed for military families and their young children to share.

Veterans Suicide Prevention Hotline

www.suicidepreventionlifeline.org/Veterans

The Department of Veterans Affairs' (VA) Veterans Health Administration as a national suicide prevention hotline to ensure veterans in emotional crisis have free, 24/7 access to trained counselors. The website includes a veterans resource locator to assist in locating crisis and mental health services at medical centers and community-based outpatient clinics in your area.

Phone: 1-800-273-TALK (800-273-8255), veterans press 1; (Spanish/Español: 888-628-9454)
24-hour Veteran Combat Call Center help line answered by combat veterans: 1-877-927-8387 (WAR-VETS).

U.S. General

Anxiety Disorders Association of America

www.adaa.org/finding-help

The Anxiety Disorders Association of America (ADAA) provides resources for support and tips for helping friends and relatives.

American Association of Suicidology
www.suicidology.org
   This national clearinghouse for information about suicide offers books and resources such as fact sheets, statistics, and public education materials. Website describes what steps to take to get help for someone thinking of committing suicide. Offers referrals to suicide survivor support groups.

5221 Wisconsin Avenue, NW
Washington, DC 20015
Phone: 202-237-2280

American Foundation for Suicide Prevention
www.afsp.org
   Provides information and support, including programs to help survivors cope with loss and a national directory of survivor support groups in U.S. states for families and friends. The website lists the warning signs that a loved one may be contemplating suicide. The list of resources includes videos, books, personal stories, and studies on suicide.

120 Wall Street
22nd Floor
New York, NY 10005
Phone: 888-333-2377 or 212-363-3500

American Psychiatric Association
www.psych.org

American Psychological Association
www.apa.org/helpcenter
   The American Psychological Association Help Center offers useful guidance on various topics related to trauma and families. Referrals to psychologist also available through the website.

Association for Behavioral and Cognitive Therapies
www.abct.org/Members/?=findtherapist&fa=FT_Form&nolm=1
   The ABCT (formerly AABT) maintains a database of therapists.

Badge of Life—Psychological Survival for Police Officers
www.badgeoflife.com
   The police volunteers at Badge of Life will help you with presentations and training seminars to create a better quality of mental health for police officers and to prevent suicide. Their board of directors consists of retired and active cops, a psychiatrist, clinical social worker, a psychiatric nurse, and major consultants in the mental health field. The website also provides information for grieving families.

Andy O'Hara, Executive Director
Badge of Life
PO Box 2203
Citrus Heights, CA 95611
Phone: 916-212-3144

Compassionate Friends

www.compassionatefriends.org

Assists families toward the positive resolution of grief following the death of a child of any age and provides information to help others be supportive.

Phone: 877-969-0010 or 630-990-0010
Fax: 630-990-0246

Gift from Within

www.giftfromwithin.org

This is a nonprofit organization dedicated to those who suffer from PTSD, those at risk for PTSD, and those who care for traumatized individuals. Includes essays, articles, poetry and art, meditations, Q&A on PTSD, podcasts, book reviews, and more.

Mental Health America (formerly known as National Mental Health Association)

www.nmha.org/go/ptsd

National Alliance on Mental Illness (NAMI)

www.nami.org

NAMI is a grassroots mental health advocacy organization dedicated to improving the lives of individuals and families affected by mental illness. NAMI offers education and support for persons afflicted with mental illness and their families.

Information Helpline: 1 (800) 950-NAMI (6264)

National Association of Social Workers

www.helpstartshere.org/find-a-social-worker

The therapist locator page for the National Association of Social Workers.

National Child Traumatic Stress Network

www.nctsn.org

Established by Congress in 2000, this unique collaboration of academic and community-based service centers is devoted to raising the standard of care and increase access to services for traumatized children and their families. Combining knowledge of child development, expertise in the full range of child traumatic experiences, and attention to cultural perspectives, the NCTSN serves as a national resource for developing and disseminating evidence-based interventions, trauma-informed services, and public and professional education.

National Coalition Against Domestic Violence
www.ncadv.org

The website contains information for making a safety plan, protecting families, and finding state and local resources to support victims of domestic violence; information on domestic violence; and links to other helpful organizations.

NCADV's Main Office
1120 Lincoln Street, Suite #1603
Denver, CO 80203
Phone: (303) 839-1852
TTY: (303) 839-8459
Fax: (303) 831-9251
E-mail: *mainoffice@ncadv.org*

National Institute of Mental Health
www.nimh.nih.gov/health/topics/post-traumatic-stress-disorder-ptsd/index.shtml

The National Women's Health Information Center
www.womenshealth.gov/faq/sexual-assault.cfm
The Sexual Assault Information Page of the U.S. federal government's source for women's health information.

Pandora's Project
www.pandys.org

Support and resources for survivors of rape and sexual abuse. Provides information, facilitates peer support, and offers assistance to male and female survivors of sexual violence and their friends and families. Sponsors the Internet's largest support community for those who have been the victim of sexual violence. Available 24 hours a day and free of charge to any survivor who has Internet access, the Pandora's Aquarium message board and chat room offer victims of sexual violence a refuge to share experiences, seek advice, and provide support. The organization also operates a free sexual assault lending library, maintains resource lists for survivors in need of face-to-face support, and organizes retreat weekends for survivors ready to take their healing one step further. Pandora's Project is managed and staffed by more than 50 survivors, all of whom are unpaid volunteers.

3109 West 50th Street, Suite #320
Minneapolis, MN 55410-2102
E-mail: *admin@pandys.org*

Rape, Abuse, and Incest National Network
www.rainn.org

RAINN carries out programs to prevent sexual assault, helps victims, and attempts to ensure that rapists are brought to justice. Its website contains statistics, counseling resources, prevention tips, and news. RAINN operates the

National Sexual Assault Hotline at 1-800-656-HOPE in partnership with 1,100 rape crisis centers across the nation, providing free, confidential advice 24/7. It also operates the National Sexual Assault Online Hotline, providing live, secure help to victims through an interface as intuitive as instant messaging.

2000 L Street NW, Suite 406
Washington, DC 20036
Phone: 202-544-3064
Fax: 202-544-3556
E-mail: *info@rainn.org*

SAMHSA's Disaster/Trauma Information Page
www.samhsa.gov/trauma/index.aspx
   From the Substance Abuse and Mental Health Services Administration (SAMHSA) website. SAMHSA is part of the U.S. Department of Health and Human Services and provides public information and referrals on mental health services. The center offers a toll-free number and crisis hotline, and people may also write for information. Free publications on a range of mental health issues are also available. SAMHSA's information specialists answer callers' questions and refer them to federal, state, or local resources for more information and help. The center offers up-to-the-minute information on issues such as prevention, treatment, and recovery services for mental illness and on subjects ranging from advocacy to suicide prevention.

PO Box 2345
Rockville, MD 20847
Phone: 800-789-2647, 240-221-4021 (international callers)
Fax: 240-221-4295
TDD: 1-866-889-2647 or 240-221-4022 (international callers)

SAMHSA's Substance Abuse Treatment Locator
findtreatment.samhsa.gov
   Find services for the general public as well as veterans.

SIDRAN Institute Help Desk
www.sidran.org
   This nationally focused nonprofit organization devoted to helping people who have experienced traumatic life events offers a referral list of therapists, as well as a fact sheet on how to choose a therapist for PTSD and dissociative disorders.

Sesame Street Parents
www.sesamestreet.org/parents
   Advice by Sesameworkshop.org about how to talk with children about tragedy, and when to seek professional help.

WebMD PTSD Information Page
www.webmd.com/anxiety-panic/guide/post-traumatic-stress-disorder
WebMD offers medical news, features, reference material, and online community programs.

International

About.com
ptsd.about.com
The PTSD & Trauma Resource Page contains a comprehensive listing of information, resources, links, and support groups on a wide array of topics related to trauma, particularly incest and child abuse.

Daily Strength
www.dailystrength.org/c/Post-Traumatic_Stress_Disorder/forum
Web-based support for a variety of concerns. This is the PTSD forum link.

David Baldwin's Trauma Information Pages
www.trauma-pages.com

International Society for Traumatic Stress Studies
www.istss.org

111 Deer Lake Road, Suite 100
Deerfield, IL 60015
Phone: 1-847-480-9028
Fax: 1-847-480-9282

PTSD Forum
www.ptsdforum.org
Aims to help PTSD sufferers and their spouses and families help themselves through others' experiences, guidance, and education.

Books

Armstrong, K., Best, S., & Domenici, P. (2005). *Courage after fire: Coping strategies for troops returning from Iraq and Afghanistan and their families.* Berkeley, CA: Ulysses Press.

Carney, C., & Manber, R. (2009). *Quiet your mind and get to sleep: Solutions to insomnia for those with depression, anxiety or chronic pain.* Oakland, CA: New Harbinger.

Davis, M., Eshelman, E. R., McKay, M., & Fanning, P. (2008). *The relaxation and stress reduction workbook* (6th ed.). Oakland, CA: New Harbinger.

Herbert, C., & Wetmore, A. (2008). *Overcoming traumatic stress: A self-help guide using cognitive behavioral techniques.* New York: Basic Books.

Jakubowski, P., & Lange, A. J. (1978). *The assertive option.* Champaign, IL: Research Press.

Kabat-Zinn, J. (1990). *Full catastrophe living: Using the wisdom of your body and mind to face stress, pain, and illness.* New York: Bantam Books.

Kabat-Zinn, J. (1994). *Wherever you go there you are: Mindfulness meditation in everyday life.* New York: Hyperion.

Matsakis, A. (2005). *In harm's way: Help for the wives of military men, police, EMTs, and firefighters.* Oakland, CA: New Harbinger.

Meyers, R. J., & Wolfe, B. L. (2003). *Getting your loved one sober: Alternatives to nagging, pleading, and threatening.* Minneapolis: Hazelden.

Moore, B. A., & Kennedy, C. H. (2010). *Wheels down: Adjusting to life after deployment.* Washington, DC: American Psychological Association.

Nay, W. R. (2010). *Overcoming anger in your relationship: How to break the cycle of arguments, put-downs, and stony silences.* New York: Guilford Press.

Paleg, K., & McKay, M. (2001). *When anger hurts your relationship: 10 simple solutions for couples who fight.* Oakland, CA: New Harbinger.

Phillips, S. B., & Kane, D. (2009). *Healing together: A couple's guide to coping with trauma and post-traumatic stress.* Oakland, CA: New Harbinger.

Rosenbloom, D., & Williams, M. B. (2010). *Life after trauma: A workbook for healing* (2nd ed.). New York: Guilford Press.

Scott, C. (2007). *Moving on after trauma: A guide for survivors, family, and friends.* East Sussex, UK: Routledge.

Sherman, M. D., & Sherman, D. M. (2005). *Finding my way: A teen's guide to living with a parent who has experienced trauma.* Edina, MN: Beavers Pond Press.

Silberman, S. (2008). *The insomnia workbook: A comprehensive guide to getting the sleep you need.* Oakland, CA: New Harbinger.

Slone, L. B., & Friedman, M. J. (2008). *After the war zone: A practical guide for returning troops and their families.* Cambridge, MA: Da Capo Press.

Smith, J. (1995). *Car accident: A practical recovery manual for drivers, passengers, and the people in their lives.* Cleveland, OH: StressPress.

Turk, D. C., & Frits, W. (2005). *The pain survival guide: How to reclaim your life.* Washington, DC: American Psychological Association.

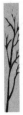

References

Albright, D. L., & Thyer, B. (2010). Does EMDR reduce posttraumatic stress disorder symptomatology in combat veterans? *Behavioral Interventions, 25*(1), 1–19.

Bradley, R., Greene, J., Russ, E., Dutra, L., & Westen, D. (2005). A multidimensional meta-analysis of psychotherapy for PTSD. *American Journal of Psychiatry, 162*(2), 214–227.

Calhoun, L. G., & Tedeschi, R. G. (2006). *Handbook of posttraumatic growth: Research and practice.* Mahwah, NJ: Erlbaum.

Campbell, R. (2008). The psychological impact of rape victims, experiences with the legal, medical, and mental health systems. *American Psychologist, 63*(8), 702–717.

Foa, E. B., Keane, T. M., Friedman, M. J., & Cohen, J. A. (2009). *Effective treatments for PTSD: Practice guidelines from the International Society for Traumatic Stress Studies* (2nd ed.). New York: Guilford Press.

Fournier, J. C., DeRubeis, R. J., Hollon, S. D., Dimidjian, S., Amsterdam, J. D., Shelton, R. C., et al. (2009). Antidepressant drug effects and depression severity: A patient-level meta-analysis. *Journal of the American Medical Association, 303*(1), 47–53.

Jakubowski, P., & Lange, A. J. (1978). *The assertive option.* Champaign, IL: Research Press.

Meichenbaum, D. (2006). Resilience and posttraumatic growth: A constructive narrative perspective. In L. G. Calhoun & R. G. Tedeschi (Eds.), *Handbook of posttraumatic growth* (pp. 355–367). Mahwah, NJ: Erlbaum.

Najavits, L. M. (2002). *Seeking safety: A treatment manual for PTSD and substance abuse.* New York: Guilford Press.

National Center for Victims of Crime & Crime Victims Research and Treatment Center. (1992). *Rape in America: A report to the nation.* Arlington, VA: National Center for Victims of Crime.

Penava, S. J., Otto, M. W., Pollack, M. H., & Rosenbaum, J. F. (1996). Current status of pharmacotherapy for PTSD: An effect size analysis of controlled studies. *Depression and Anxiety, 4*(5), 240–242.

Ponniah, K., & Hollon, S. D. (2009). Empirically supported psychological treatments for adult acute stress disorder and posttraumatic stress disorder: A review. *Depression and Anxiety, 26*(12), 1086–1109.

Powers, M. B., Halpern, J. M., Ferenschak, M. P., Gillihan, S. J., & Foa, E. B. (2010). A meta-analytic review of prolonged exposure for posttraumatic stress disorder. *Clinical Psychology Review, 30*(6), 635–641.

Raskind, M. A. (2009). Pharmacologic treatment of PTSD. In P. J. Shiromani, T. M. Keane, & J. E. LeDoux (Eds.), *Post-traumatic stress disorder: Basic science and clinical practice* (pp. 337–361). New York: Humana Press.

Ready, D. J., Thomas, K. R., Worley, V., Backscheider, A. G., Harvey, L. A. C., Baltzell, D., et al. (2008). A field test of group-based exposure therapy with 102 veterans with war-related posttraumatic stress disorder. *Journal of Traumatic Stress, 21*(2), 150–157.

Resnick, H., Kilpatrick, D. G., Dansky, B. S., Saunders, B. E., & Best, C. (1993). Prevalence of civilian trauma and posttraumatic stress disorder in a representative national sample of women. *Journal of Consulting and Clinical Psychology, 61*(6), 984–991.

Rothbaum, B. O., Foa, E. B., Riggs, D. S., Murdock, T., & Walsh, W. (2006). A prospective examination of post-traumatic stress disorder in rape victims. *Journal of Tramatic Stress, 5*(3), 455–475.

Schubert, S., & Lee, C. W. (2009). Adult PTSD and its treatment with EMDR: A review of controversies, evidence, and theoretical knowledge. *Journal of EMDR Practice and Research, 3*(3), 117–132.

Taft, C. T., Weatherill, R. P., Woodward, H. E., Pinto, L. A., Watkins, L. E., Miller, M. W., et al. (2009). Intimate partner and general aggression perpetration among combat veterans presenting to a posttraumatic stress disorder clinic. *American Journal of Orthopsychiatry, 79*(4), 461–468.

Tewksbury, R. (2007). Effects of sexual assaults on men: Physical, mental and sexual consequences. *International Journal of Men's Health, 6*(1), 22–35.

Widom, C. S. (1999). Posttraumatic stress disorder in abused and neglected children grown up. *American Journal of Psychiatry, 156*(8), 1223–1229.

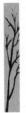

Index

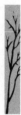

About the Authors

Claudia Zayfert, PhD, a clinical psychologist, is an internationally renowned expert in cognitive-behavioral therapy who has been helping trauma survivors overcome posttraumatic stress for over 20 years. Dr. Zayfert is coauthor of *Cognitive-Behavioral Therapy for PTSD: A Case Formulation Approach*. She is Associate Professor of Psychiatry at Dartmouth Medical School and Director of the Anxiety Disorders Service at Dartmouth–Hitchcock Medical Center in Lebanon, New Hampshire, where she teaches and conducts clinical research on trauma-related problems.

Jason C. DeViva, PhD, is a clinical psychologist in the Veterans Affairs Connecticut Health Care System, where he works extensively with veterans returning from Iraq and Afghanistan. Dr. DeViva is on the faculties of the University of Connecticut School of Medicine and Yale School of Medicine. He has worked in the field of posttraumatic stress for more than a decade, conducting research, providing outreach and education, and treating civilians and veterans with posttraumatic stress disorder and related problems.